THE
EVERYTHING
GUIDE TO
AYURVEDA

Dear Reader,

I'm so glad to have this opportunity to support you and your family as you explore the science of life called Ayurveda.

Before I found Ayurveda, I was searching for answers to simple questions: What should I eat, what exercise is best for me long-term, can I balance work and relaxation? With all the information on the Internet, in commercials, and in magazines, it was hard for me to find a trustworthy, natural, and practical way to health. I didn't want a quick fix; I wanted to learn how to enjoy life without catching annual colds, suffering from seasonal allergies, and developing chronic headaches. And, most of all, I wanted to do it naturally and in a way that could support me through my later years of life. Ayurveda has the answers, and it's been in practice for more than 5,000 years!

Now, I am thrilled to offer you this doorway into the vast science of Ayurveda. It's a system of health that allows you to learn more about who you truly are and what you personally need. May the words in this book inspire you to enjoy the road to a naturally healthy, happy, and long life.

Namaste,

Heidi E. Spear

Welcome to the EVERYTHING® Series!

These handy, accessible books give you all you need to tackle a difficult project, gain a new hobby, comprehend a fascinating topic, prepare for an exam, or even brush up on something you learned back in school but have since forgotten.

You can choose to read an Everything® book from cover to cover or just pick out the information you want from our four useful boxes: e-questions, e-facts, e-quotes, and e-ssentials.

We give you everything you need to know on the subject, but throw in a lot of fun stuff along the way, too.

We now have more than 400 Everything® books in print, spanning such wide-ranging categories as weddings, pregnancy, cooking, music instruction, foreign language, crafts, pets, New Age, and so much more. When you're done reading them all, you can finally say you know Everything®!

QUESTION

Answers to
common questions

FACT

Important snippets
of information

QUOTE

Words of wisdom from
experts in the field

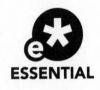

ESSENTIAL

Quick
handy tips

PUBLISHER Karen Cooper

DIRECTOR OF ACQUISITIONS AND INNOVATION Paula Munier

MANAGING EDITOR, EVERYTHING® SERIES Lisa Laing

COPY CHIEF Casey Ebert

ASSISTANT PRODUCTION EDITOR Melanie Cordova

ACQUISITIONS EDITOR Kate Powers

SENIOR DEVELOPMENT EDITOR Brett Palana-Shanahan

EDITORIAL ASSISTANT Ross Weisman

EVERYTHING® SERIES COVER DESIGNER Erin Alexander

LAYOUT DESIGNERS Erin Dawson, Michelle Roy Kelly, Elisabeth Lariviere, Denise Wallace

Visit the entire Everything® series at *www.everything.com*

THE EVERYTHING®

GUIDE TO AYURVEDA

Improve your health, develop your inner energy,
and find balance in your life

Heidi E. Spear

Foreword by Hilary Garivaltis,
Dean of the Kripalu School of Ayurveda

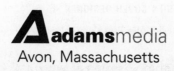

Aadamsmedia
Avon, Massachusetts

To my mother, Sandie; my father, Stan;
and my brother, Scott

An Everything® Series Book.
Everything® and everything.com® are registered trademarks of F+W Media, Inc.

Published by Adams Media, a division of F+W Media, Inc.
57 Littlefield Street, Avon, MA 02322 U.S.A.
www.adamsmedia.com

Contains material adapted and abridged from *The Everything® Guide to
Chakra Healing* by Heidi E. Spear, copyright © 2011 by F+W Media, Inc.;
ISBN 10: 1-4405-2584-6; ISBN 13: 978-1-4405-2584-1.

Masala Recipes in Chapter 6: © 2011 Jonathan Dahari-Lanciano
Standing Meditation in Chapter 8 and the yoga and breathwork
sequences in Chapters 10 and 12: © 2011 Janna Delgado
Recipes for Halva Treats and Digestive Chew and yoga and breathwork sequences
in Chapters 8 and 20: © 2011 Sudha Carolyn Lundeen, RN, RYT-500
Recipes for Soba Noodles and Sun-Dried Tomatoes, Lunch Burrito, Indian Chickpeas, Gourmet Squash,
Simply Baked Salmon, Wild Rice Pecan Pilaf, Root Veggie Bake, Hummus, Lemon Dill Potatoes, Ginger
Lentil Spread, Peanut Sauce, Fun Dessert Crispies, and
Oatmeal Chocolate Cookies: © 2011 Nourish Your Light, All Rights Reserved.

ISBN 10: 1-4405-2996-5
ISBN 13: 978-1-4405-2996-2
eISBN 10: 1-4405-3045-9
eISBN 13: 978-1-4405-3045-6

Printed in the United States of America.

10 9 8 7 6 5 4 3 2 1

Library of Congress Cataloging-in-Publication Data
is available from the publisher.

This book is intended as general information only, and should not be used to diagnose or treat any health condition. In light of the complex, individual, and specific nature of health problems, this book is not intended to replace professional medical advice. The ideas, procedures, and suggestions in this book are intended to supplement, not replace, the advice of a trained medical professional. Consult your physician before adopting any of the suggestions in this book, as well as about any condition that may require diagnosis or medical attention. The author and publisher disclaim any liability arising directly or indirectly from the use of this book.

Many of the designations used by manufacturers and sellers to distinguish their products are claimed as trademarks. Where those designations appear in this book and Adams Media was aware of a trademark claim, the designations have been printed with initial capital letters.

This book is available at quantity discounts for bulk purchases.
For information, please call 1-800-289-0963.

Contents

Acknowledgments

A book is so much more than the knowledge it aims to pass on. A book holds the energy of all those who contribute to its production and make it possible for everyone to do her part. I send so much gratitude to everyone at Adams Media who worked on this book. Specifically, I appreciate Kate Powers for her patience and expertise in guiding this project from inception to completion. I am grateful to the editorial team at Adams Media and to Hilary Garivaltis for writing the foreword.

It's been such a pleasure to work with colleagues who contributed knowledge and expertise to this project. Thanks so much to Sudha Carolyn Lundeen for her valuable work: the vata breathwork and yoga sections, as well as a couple of not-to-be-missed recipes (her halva balls and digestive chew). Janna Delgado's breathwork and yoga sequences for pitta and kapha are creatively inspired, just like her yoga classes. I'm so grateful to be able to include her voice in those sections of the book, as well as in the section that describes a standing meditation. Jonathan Dahari-Lanciano shares his mastery of spice masalas, which add balancing and satisfying tastes to meals at any time of day. Danny Arguetty's personal experience with Ayurveda shines in the writing and recipes he contributed. His culinary delights are simple to make, nourishing, and fun to eat. Patricia Lemer also contributed healthy, flavorful recipes, showcasing her ability to choose meals that are comforting and deeply nourishing. I am also grateful to my mother for sharing her sought-after recipe for perfect pecans! Thanks to Sarajean Rudman for her important contributions that form much of the Top 10 list at the start of this book. Also, thank you to Sadie Cunningham, whose writing gives a glimpse into what makes Ayurvedic bodywork unique, particularly as a restorative and balancing treatment. Sadie has a gift for transmitting healing energy, which is apparent even in her written word.

This book could not have happened without the gracious support of Kelley Johnson Boyd, whose enthusiastic encouragement and sensitivity toward the writing process showed up in numerous ways. Thank you also to Karen Li, Beth Haydon Bodan, Sally Segerstrom, Cristie Newhart, Liz Walz, Joshua Needleman, and Hallie Deen for your unwavering support during the writing process.

The Top 10 Ayurvedic Tips for Healthy Living

1. Let the first thing you drink in the morning be a glass of warm water (add some lemon juice if you'd like).

2. Give yourself an oil massage in the morning before you shower or bathe: it feels good and helps the blood and lymph circulate through the body.

3. Get outside for a walk and breathe in fresh air every day.

4. Each time you eat, take your time and enjoy the nourishing food.

5. Have your biggest meal at lunchtime.

6. Sip warm water throughout the day to stay hydrated and support digestive fire.

7. As an alternative to coffee, for an energy boost without caffeine that can also help reduce stress, make tulsi tea.

8. Always buy the freshest produce you can, local and organic when possible.

9. Take time before bed to wind down from your day by spending time relaxing or spending time with friends or family.

10. Enjoy creating balance in your life as you make choices according to this observation in nature: opposites balance, like increases like.

Foreword

Ayurveda, often translated as "the Science of Life," can also be considered "universal knowledge." More simply put, it is our "owner's manual" that teaches us how to keep ourselves running well from birth to death. Just like other creatures are wired into natural rhythms in nature such as hibernation or migration patterns, the human being, or homo sapien, is wired with particular rhythms as well. No one can escape this fact. The more we align with our natural rhythms, the more balanced and harmonious we are, and as an extension of our existence, the more harmonious we are, the more harmonious the world becomes. These premises sit strongly in the system of Ayurvedic Medicine and guide every aspect of existence.

All "traditional" systems of medicine are rooted in the true study of nature. Ayurveda is one of the unique systems that has been actually practicing and codifying this knowledge for over 5,000 years. This vast and elegant knowledge has stood the test of time and continues to be relevant in this modern age. What I have learned to love so much about Ayurveda is that I can find answers so easily to some of the most complicated scenarios and that the system itself teaches us through very simple means to be observant and how to make the best choices for the best outcomes.

Ayurveda teaches us the tools of living well and how to correct brewing imbalances through simple changes to daily routines, food choices, exercise, and through use of natural herbal formulas or treatment protocols. Ayurveda is not only a science but a complete medical system based on sound principles of science, and as a system of medicine spanning thousands of years, it not only carries the knowledge base forward rooted in science, but it also can verify its effectiveness through its repeated applications and verifiable results that have been "tried and true" for all these many years. There is great comfort in this for me as a practitioner and teacher of this amazing science.

I have been studying for over a dozen years and have only scratched the surface of the complexities of Mother Nature, and at the same time I have also been shown time and time again how easy change can be and how effective simple alterations to our diet and lifestyle (the cornerstone of Ayurveda) can reverse and often completely change pathologies that create disharmony and ill health.

I am often heard saying, "It is the simple things that make the biggest difference," as well as "What you align with each day is more important than the occasional variances in life." A simple guide is often all we need. Try not to make life and harmony more complicated than it is. Remember to keep it simple and always check in with yourself and ask, is this supporting me or not?

The Everything® Guide to Ayurveda is a great place to start your journey. It will help you begin to find your own balance through the lens and guidance of Ayurveda.

Enjoy and be well!
Hilary Garivaltis
Dean of the Kripalu School of Ayurveda

Introduction

ARE YOU SEARCHING FOR a simple and authentic manual on how to live a healthy and vibrant life? Would you like a natural and easy-to-understand guide that explains how to nourish yourself and your family so you all can be healthier and happier? Do you wish that someone could give you suggestions about how to relax your mind and body, even though you live a busy life? If you answer "yes" to these questions, you may have finally found the guide you're looking for: it's the holistic system of health called Ayurveda.

Ayurveda is Sanskrit for "the science of life." If you've never heard of Ayurveda, don't worry that the name seems unfamiliar. This extensive system of health was conceived long before English was a common language. This health system—which explains how to use whole foods, herbs, and spices as sustenance for health and longevity—originated in India more than 5,000 years ago. Now, it's gaining popularity worldwide for its natural, holistic, and time-tested wisdom.

One of the many reasons Ayurveda is so attractive is that it's profound and practical. As you read the wisdom of Ayurveda, you'll feel its deep roots in time and tradition, and at the same time you'll see how relevant it is to your life today.

Many in the West, including doctors, are very interested in learning about Ayurveda, as well as other alternative and complementary medicines. People are beginning to realize that even though Western medicine can save someone's life, it alone cannot create deep, long-lasting comfortable health and longevity. One reason for this is because traditional Western medicine focuses only on the specific location of discomfort that you feel, or a site-specific diagnosis.

For complete health and healing, all aspects of you (mind, body, and spirit) must be considered for all conditions—from a common cold to a heart attack. Ayurveda is a holistic approach that observes all aspects of who you are and what's going on in your life. Your Ayurvedic specialist will want to learn about you as an individual. After she listens to you and performs her examination, she can determine your constitution and your present condition. Then, she can explain what you need in order to create balance, health, and happiness in your life.

According to Ayurveda, you have all the qualities of the natural elements (ether, air, fire, water, and earth) within you. Qualities such as hot, cold, smooth, rough, light, and heavy exist in nature, and they exist inside of you to varying degrees. Ayurveda uses the terminology of elemental qualities to determine your specific constitution and present condition. Once you know your individual constitution and the state of the elements in you, from there you will be able to tell which foods, exercises, and other life choices will best support your mind, body, and spirit. There are always plenty of options for every constitution!

This book will give you a strong foundational understanding of Ayurveda whether you already see a specialist or not. After determining your constitution, you can use this book as a handy reference, full of reminders, recipes, exercises, and support for you and your family.

In the following pages, you will learn the basics of Ayurveda, its history, and how it can bring health and happiness to you and your family. You'll find specific ways to nourish yourself and your children: body, mind, and spirit. You will see how being healthy can be a fun, nurturing, and creative experience as you try the various recipes, yoga for each constitutional type, and simple home remedies. You will learn how to be healthy with preventive measures, supporting your immunity on a daily basis, and you'll learn about special therapeutic modalities, such as Ayurvedic bodywork and chakra balancing.

Ayurvedic wisdom will help you provide great meals and activities for your family. You may have noticed by now that no two children (in fact, no two people) are the same. Using Ayurveda as your guide, you'll be able to evaluate how your children look, act, feel, and digest their food so you can determine how to help them stay healthy. Ayurveda will help you account for the individual needs of each person to create health, harmony, and happiness in the home.

If you're looking for a natural, compassionate, and extensive science to explain how to live life and to age with health, radiance, and ease, then Ayurveda is the exquisite and natural lifestyle for you.

CHAPTER 1

What Is Ayurveda?

Ayurveda is a holistic, natural system of health, originating in India more than 5,000 years ago. Perhaps the oldest extant medical system in the world, Ayurveda's teachings are timeless. Now, when looking for natural, holistic, and safe ways to create health for themselves and their families, people in the West are interested in Ayurveda for its vast knowledge and effective treatments. Ayurveda offers remedies for illness and is designed as a preventive medicine that supports consistent health and longevity.

A Complete Medical System

Ayurveda is a complete medical system. It treats the whole person as an integrated being: body, mind, and spirit. Ayurveda is a comprehensive medical system that includes: surgery, psychotherapy, pediatrics, gynecology, obstetrics, ophthalmology, geriatrics, ear/nose/throat, and general medicine. All of these branches are subsumed in the holistic practice of Ayurveda, which takes into consideration all aspects of your life, and employs a variety of healing modalities to support your health and thriving day by day, year by year.

Nonspecialized Treatment

Ayurveda doesn't specialize, which means it doesn't focus on healing just one organ or one symptom at a time. Your Ayurvedic practitioner will be interested in your history and all of your physical symptoms (headache, stomachache, sore back, etc.). She will ask you a variety of questions and perform a physical examination. Her examination helps her understand what is causing you to experience uncomfortable symptoms and disease.

Then, she will give you recommendations to treat the symptoms and bring you back into balance, primarily through lifestyle and diet. The recommendations will be nourishing for your body, mind, and spirit. As you eat the foods and herbs she recommends, savor the tastes, scents, and textures. Support the healing power of these herbs and foods with trust in their healing potential. Your thoughts, energy, and beliefs will help your healing process. In addition, the appropriate foods, herbs, and lifestyle changes give your body, mind, and spirit the support to heal.

Once you are feeling well again, your Ayurvedic practitioner will give you recommendations to maintain balance, which is the condition for optimal health. When in balance, you'll notice what it feels like to be enjoying good health and immunity. Your symptoms will disappear, you'll feel less irritable, you'll think more clearly, you'll catch fewer colds (if any), and you can even reduce or stop suffering from seasonal allergies. You'll feel well and be able to enjoy your life more.

When you start to get sick, if you choose not to make changes in your diet and lifestyle and instead only take allopathic drugs for the symptoms, it's likely that your symptoms will worsen and/or recur. In Ayurveda, the idea is to create harmony in your mind, body, and spirit so your body can support its own healing and become well enough to discourage recurring symptoms and the development of disease.

QUESTION

What is the benefit of Ayurveda as a holistic practice, one that doesn't specialize?
As a holistic practice, Ayurveda creates overall health, recognizing that body, mind, and spirit are interrelated. So, its goal is twofold: to alleviate the discomfort of something such as a headache, stomachache, or cold, and to bring you into balance to prevent those symptoms from recurring and worsening.

Your body wants to be well, and it's designed to function in harmony with the natural world. To create health, your body must be able to perform its vital functions, which include the absorption of vitamins and minerals, and the elimination of toxins. Rather than just suggesting a quick fix, Ayurveda gives you the tools to create a state of harmony in your body and mind so that your body can perform its required functions to keep you healthy.

Each Moment Counts

Ayurveda is a way of living. It's about being healthy from moment to moment, day by day. As you wake up in the morning, as you eat your meals, as you schedule in time for exercise and play, Ayurveda teaches you to consider what nourishes your mind, body, and spirit.

FACT

What you eat, what you watch on TV, how much time you spend exchanging the energy of love with others—everything you do, say, think, and feel has an impact on your body, mind, and energy system. There isn't one thing you do that doesn't affect all of you, and you can make moment-to-moment choices for equilibrium.

Each moment gives you the opportunity to make a choice. In each moment you can choose to do something that helps create balance in you or that may bring you out of balance. Ayurveda gives you knowledge about yourself and your relationship to the external world so that you can make informed choices moment by moment, meal by meal, day by day, and season by season.

One Choice at a Time

Your health will improve as you make one choice at a time. You have choices—what to eat, what to think, what to wear, when to exercise, whom to hang out with, how to manage your reactions. If it seems as though you don't have time or energy to make new choices, think about this: you can make one small change at a time. And, notice how it makes you feel. Then, decide if you'd like to incorporate another change. Go at your own pace. Keep remembering, you are the one who decides how to take care of yourself. It's up to you. Ayurveda offers natural, simple guidelines to bring you into a life of balance for longevity, health, and vitality.

QUESTION

Will I have to follow a rigid and strict diet?
Ayurveda is about balance. You will learn which foods are best at which times of year. You can enjoy any food in moderation, and if you choose something that isn't the best for your system, you will know how to re-create balance. Over time, you may actually want to avoid foods that right now you think you can't live without.

As a **whole medical system**, a nonspecializing system, Ayurveda treats your entire being. The diet and lifestyle changes it suggests are simple and basic, and "one step at a time" is a great way to approach it if it feels like too much at once. As a science, Ayurveda actually makes sense, and you'll be able to notice when you're sliding out of balance. Then, you can turn to Ayurvedic guidance to keep yourself healthy year-round. You can also have fun with it—customizing recipes and enjoying its natural and life-affirming recommendations. You'll see, it's a whole new way to view health—in a positive way that supports the lifestyle your body, mind, and spirit desire.

The History of Ayurveda

Ayurveda is Sanskrit for "the science of life." *Ayur* means "life," and veda means "to know," or "knowledge." So, Ayurveda is the knowledge of what it is to be living, of how to live healthily and in harmony with this planet and all that is. More than 5,000 years ago, **rishis**, or seers of truth, passed down the knowledge of Ayurveda to only their students as an oral tradition. Now, Ayurveda has become a part of the consciousness of mainstream Western lifestyle.

The Beginnings of Ayurveda

In a way very different from many modern Western medical discoveries, Ayurveda didn't originate in laboratories or research centers. More than 5,000 years ago, while in meditative states, rishis in India began to understand the nature of life, health, and longevity that has come to be what we call Ayurveda, the science of life. This, combined with more than 5,000 years of observing the systems inherent in the natural world, forms a study of the complex nature of our existence. One of the many gifts of Ayurveda is the vast knowledge of the plant world, which has helped create one of the most fine-tuned pharmacopoeias of natural medicines the world has known.

FACT

For millennia, in India they've known that meditation and present-moment awareness are vehicles for tapping in to the wisdom of the universe. When you meditate, becoming still and quiet, you open to knowledge and wisdom beyond your studies. Knowledge is of the mind; wisdom is of the heart. Combining learning through study and receiving through meditation reveals the wisdom of living.

More than 2,000 years ago much of Ayurveda's wisdom was transcribed into Sanskrit. Many of those texts are still around today. Ayurvedic specialists learn from the wisdom of these texts and from the wisdom of practitioners who combine that knowledge with their proven experience in Ayurveda and **allopathic**, or traditional Western, medicine.

You Have the Same Elements as the Eternal Cosmos

One of the philosophers of this age, Kapila, is credited with the philosophy of creation known as **Samkya** from the roots *sat*, meaning "truth," and *kyah*, meaning "to know." This "knowledge of truth" is the foundation of Ayurveda. According to Samkya philosophy, before physical matter existed there were two eternal forces: consciousness that is pure awareness, called **Purusha**, and a force of creativity/action called **Prakruti**. Purusha, awareness, is considered the male energy of the universe. It is pure awareness. It is the universal intelligence and consciousness that just is. Prakruti is considered the female energy of the universe, which is awareness plus choice and the desire for creation. It is from the energy of Prakruti that the universe, and each human being, has come into existence.

ESSENTIAL

Ayurveda's nontheistic creation story is compatible with theistic beliefs. If you believe in a creator, it's also possible to incorporate the realization that you are made of the same elements that you experience outside. Samkya philosophy explains that your physical and energetic bodies are composed of the same elements as the natural world.

Samkya explains that each human being is a microcosm of the macrocosm (the universe). Each person's physical makeup is a combination of the five elements of the universe. Everyone is individual in his constitution, and he is always in relationship with the energy and elements outside of himself. So, Ayurveda looks at health in terms of the individual's constitution and how to keep that in balance with the changing external elements.

Your Relationship to the Cosmos

Here is the story of creation according to the rishis who realized Samkya philosophy: Before the creation of life on earth, there existed two eternal cosmic forces: Purusha (pure awareness) and Prakruti (creative energy). Everything that is created comes from Prakruti, and Purusha is the eternal witness, with no participation in creation.

Prakruti is energy that contains the three **gunas**, or attributes: **sattva** (creative potential), **tamas** (inertia or destructive potential), and **rajas** (movement/kinetic force), in balance.

One by One, the Elements Formed

From Prakruti, the force of creation, the soundless vibration "aum" began to stir. "Aum" is said to be the first energetic vibration from which all else is born. All matter is energy at its basic unit, and "aum" is the first vibration of energy.

The vibration "aum" had to be vibrating somewhere. It was vibrating in space; that's how the rishis realized the element ether. When the element of ether began to move, it created air, the element of movement. As air began to move, it created friction, which creates heat, the element of fire. Fire has the property of transformation. Because of fire's transforming property it caused elements of ether to liquefy into water and coalesce into matter, earth. From the earth, all living matter is created, grows, and returns. This includes all the food that is nourishing to you, the water you drink, and vitamins and minerals you get from the air you breathe and the sunshine you soak up. You are of the elements, and you thrive and grow based on your relationship to them. Living in harmony with the elements keeps you healthy, youthful, and balanced. Ayurveda explains simple, natural, and fun ways to achieve this balance.

Ayurveda for the English-Speaking World

Once only available to those indigenous to India, Ayurveda now is available to the English-speaking world through various textbooks, guides, and cookbooks. In addition, there are schools of Ayurveda, where students learn through study and practice about the ancient art of Ayurveda and Ayurvedic consulting. In addition, the National Institutes of Health (NIH) includes Ayurveda among the complementary health systems it researches. The site for the National Center for Complementary and Alternative Medicine (NCCAM) is *http://nccam.nih.gov*.

In addition to being able to learn about Ayurveda through books and schools, there are workshops and websites with information and products to support your Ayurvedic lifestyle. See Appendix B for additional resources, including websites and further reading.

Your Constitution, the Doshas

Ayurveda assesses your state of being and the state of the natural world in terms of three basic principles, or doshas. The doshas are vata, pitta, and kapha. Vata dosha is a combination of the elements of ether and air, pitta is a combination of fire and water, and kapha is both water and earth elements. According to Ayurveda, your personal type, your constitution, is described by how these doshas were set in you when you were conceived.

▼ 1.1: DOSHAS AND THE ELEMENTS

Dosha	Element 1	Element 2
Vata	ether	air
Pitta	fire	water
Kapha	water	earth

All the doshas and elements are a part of you. Some people are **tri-doshic**, which means their constitution is vata-pitta-kapha. Most people are what is called "dual doshic," with two doshas sharing a higher percentage proportionally. So, the other configurations of constitutional types can be vata-pitta, vata-kapha, or pitta-kapha. To nuance a bit further one may carry a stronger proportion of one of these so there are also these last three combinations reversed to appear as pitta-vata, kapha-vata, or kapha-pitta.

FACT

The word *dosha* has two meanings. Dosha shows up in the ancient texts as the way of naming the three principles (vata, pitta, kapha). Vata, pitta, and kapha, when in balance, are the actual tissues and components of your body (dhatus). When vata, pitta, or kapha is imbalanced, dosha can also mean "impure," i.e., "vata is dosha."

Your original constitution is called your **prakruti**. Your Ayurvedic practitioner can figure out your prakruti by pulse diagnosis, and you can learn to tell which doshas are active in you once you learn which qualities are associated with each element and how to notice them in yourself. Month to month, and even hour by hour, you may notice changes in how you feel the doshas are at work inside of you. When you are out of balance, the relationship of vata-pitta-kapha in you is called your **vikruti**. For health, you want to be in balance, which means that the relationship of vata-pitta-kapha is balanced in you in the same way it was when you were born. Various lifestyle and dietary habits can bring you out of balance, and you will learn to notice when that is happening and how to steer yourself back toward balance.

The Qualities in Nature

Each dosha is described as a combination of two elements, and each element is described according to its qualities. Ayurveda lists twenty observable qualities. These qualities are expressed as ten sets of opposites: hot/cold, oily/dry, rough/smooth (slimy), heavy/light, soft/hard, static/mobile, cloudy/clear, gross/subtle, slow/sharp, liquid/solid (dense). Table 1.2 shows how Ayurveda describes each dosha and its qualities.

▼ **1.2: THE DOSHAS AND THEIR QUALITIES**

Dosha	Associated Qualities
Vata	dry, light, cold, rough, subtle, mobile, clear
Pitta	hot, sharp, light, liquid, mobile, oily
Kapha	heavy, slow, dull, cold, oily, liquid, smooth, dense, soft, static, gross, solid

Table 1.2 shows the qualities associated with each dosha, and soon these will become familiar to you. For example, "solid" is typically associated with kapha because kapha has the element of earth, which is a solid, grounding force. When you feel securely solid in your life, that is a quality of kapha in you. As you learn more about Ayurveda and start observing qualities in yourself and in nature, you may wonder which qualities go with which dosha, and that's understandable. While you are beginning to practice Ayurveda, it will help to keep these tables handy for reference. You can use both your reasoning skills and these tables to help remember which qualities are associated with which elements and doshas. And, as you do, it will become second nature for you to notice qualities in yourself, and associate those qualities to a particular element.

Why is it important to begin to associate qualities with the elements and doshas? It's foundational to the practice of Ayurveda to see yourself and the world around you in terms of the elements because the way to create health, according to Ayurveda, is to support the balance of the elements. When in balance, the elements should support the healthy flow of energy, fluids, and nutrients in the body. Your constitution, set at birth, is a particular balance of the elements in you that reflects your own unique nature. Each individual will have slightly different elemental proportions. Maintaining your unique nature and balance of these elements is the state of health for you and the state in which you will be well and live a long, healthy life. It is common to talk about the constitutional types through the language of the doshas, but it is important to see the types more properly through the concept of the elements. For the purposes of simplicity you can begin to identify body types through this paradigm: vata as ether and air, pitta as fire and water, and kapha as water and earth.

How to Recognize the Qualities in You

The following checklists are examples of how you can begin to notice how vata, pitta, and kapha are showing up in you. These checklists are to help you start to get the idea of how to observe yourself in terms of the qualities. These brief checklists are not to be used for diagnosis. They are here to give you a sense of what kinds of behaviors and patterns you'll be observing in yourself as you begin to understand your state of health according to the doshas.

OBSERVING VATA

- ❑ Do you talk quickly and often?
- ❑ Do you often feel anxious?
- ❑ Are you constipated?
- ❑ Are you more comfortable seeing the big picture rather than the small details?
- ❑ Do you easily feel connected to spiritual and energetic existence?

These questions help you determine if vata is working strongly in you. Talking quickly and often and feeling anxious have the "mobile" or "movement" quality of vata. If you're constipated, that points to the dry quality of vata. And if you tend to be more comfortable seeing the larger picture in life instead of focusing on small details, that shows the spacious/ether quality of vata. If you easily and comfortably tap in to the spiritual and creative worlds, that connection is an expression of the subtle, ethereal quality of vata. There are numerous ways to notice vata, and these are just some examples so you can understand how to notice the qualities in your behavior, mental state, and biological functions.

OBSERVING PITTA

❑ Are you able to effectively and efficiently complete tasks?
❑ Are you quick to anger?
❑ Are you highly critical of yourself and others?
❑ Are you usually hot, even when others are neutral or cold?
❑ Are you fanatical in your spiritual, religious, or nonreligious stance?

If you answered "yes" to any of these questions, you are noticing the signs of pitta in you. Just from this checklist, you aren't making a diagnosis or judgment about whether it's balanced in you or overactive. This checklist is introducing you to some of the ways to notice pitta. If you answered "yes" to any of these questions, then you are seeing pitta as noticeable in you.

Being able to effectively and efficiently complete tasks shows the "sharp" quality of the pitta mind and the fiery quality of pitta in action. If you are quick to anger and become critical, that points to the fiery and mobile qualities of pitta. If you are usually hot, even when others around you are not, that shows the hot qualities of pitta. And if you are fanatical in your relationship to spirit or adamant about your stance against the possibility of spirit, that also points to the fiery pitta energy. Remember, pitta is the dosha associated with fire.

OBSERVING KAPHA

❑ Do you gain weight easily and have difficulty losing it?
❑ Most of the year, is it hard for you to get moving?
❑ Are you prone to depression?
❑ Is your sleep heavy and long lasting?
❑ Are you loyal to your friends and loved ones?

The above checklist helps you acclimate to noticing the qualities of kapha. Kapha is a grounded, gross (as opposed to subtle) dosha. Being of earth it is hard, steady, and solid. Because of this, it's a stabilizing and nurturing force of life. Ways you may notice it in you could be that you have a larger frame and gain weight easily. You may have trouble intiating movement or projects because "mobility" is a quality associated with vata and pitta, not kapha. If you're prone to depression it could be a sign of the dense and dull qualities of kapha. If your sleep is heavy and long, that shows static and slow or lethargic qualities. And your loyalty to friends shows that solid, soft side of kapha.

How to Create Balance

To achieve a state of balance, which leads to health, these are the three principles you'll keep in mind:

- Your state of being and everything you see, touch, taste, hear, and feel can be described in terms of qualities listed in Table 1.2.
- Like increases like.
- Opposites balance.

Creating health in Ayurveda means creating balance. You will be able to adjust your diet, type of exercise, and other factors in your life to help you stay in balance throughout the various times of day, various seasons, and various times of life. Being in balance supports your biological functions, your psychological equilibrium, and your youthful spirit.

The Science of Life

Ayurveda is called the science of life. This way of life supports your getting healthy, staying healthy, and enjoying your life with youthfulness in body, mind, and spirit. Through this science of life, you will observe yourself, your family, your loved ones, and the natural world in terms of qualities. You will be able to use these observations to realize how to bring yourself and your life into balance. You'll renew your relationship to the world outside you, knowing what you need to do in response to the changing times of day, weather patterns, seasons, and years of your life so that you stay healthy.

You Are All That Is

When the rishis realized Ayurveda, they realized that all life is connected, and that health is based on recognizing this wholeness and interconnectedness. Your health is based on your recognition that you are a whole being—body, mind, and spirit—and that your existence is in relationship to all that is.

According to Ayurveda, you are both individual and a part of the entire fabric of existence. The way the elements were arranged in you at your conception makes you unique and individual. The precise choices you will make to balance yourself will differ from what your parents, your friends, and your children need to do for balance. This is because everyone is unique. At the same time, you and your loved ones are all part of the same tapestry of life. You, the sun, the moon, the flowers, the earth, your animal friends, and all beings are exchanging the same energy. You are all affected by the elements in nature, and you all have those elements at work inside of you. Because everyone and everything is connected, you are not separate from all that is.

Health Is a Dance

Staying in balance is like dancing in relationship with what's going on around you. First, you learn to notice how the doshas are in you: observe and assess the workings of your mind, body, and spirit in the moment. Once you assess how you are according to the doshas, then you know how you'll be showing up on the dance floor today. Next, note the qualities of the season and what else is going on in your external world that is beyond your control: the environment of your job, the number of to-dos you have, etc. Think in terms of the observable qualities in Table 1.2. Creating health is choreographing the dance of life so that you create harmony, beauty, and fluidity with what is inside and out moment to moment. As the music changes, you change your step. Remember, like increases like, and opposites balance as you gracefully bounce, jitterbug, and waltz with the days and seasons of life.

Peppermint is a wonderful herb for balance in summertime. If you grow it outside or buy it fresh, try smelling it (without ingesting) and notice the cooling effect on your emotions and mental state. Your sense of smell is the only sense pathway that goes straight to the limbic system—the part of the brain that experiences emotions.

To maintain your agility in the dance of life, create opposite where it's needed for balance. Take the example of someone who is pitta. If you are predominantly pitta, then your tendency is to be strong in the element of fire. Some of the qualities of pitta's fire are hot, sharp, and mobile. If you notice today you are feeling hot, irritable, and quick to anger, you will want to avoid things that will raise your heat even higher. The dance you will do for your health is to turn away from heating activities and spicy food, and glide toward places where the temperature is cooler. You'll wear light clothes and choose foods that have cooling properties. If you can avoid confrontations today, do. If you can't avoid hard conversations today, try to have a lighter attitude and intend for easeful conversations. Change your expectation, and perhaps change the outcome.

What Ayurveda Is Not

Because Ayurveda is making its way from East to West, it's possible for the modern reader to approach Ayurveda with preconceived ideas that are misconceptions rather than coming to the ideas with an open heart and mind. Be open to the wisdom of Ayurveda and see if it resonates with what makes sense to you deep down.

Ayurveda Is Not a Religion

Ayurveda takes into consideration your body, mind, and spirit because they are all connected. What does it mean to take into consideration your spirit or your relationship to spirituality? The truth of your existence is that you are in relationship with the entire universe. When you go outside in the sunshine, you can feel that you have a response to that energy. When it's cold out, you have responses that are different from your responses to when it's hot outside—you have mental, physical, and energetic responses.

You are made up of atoms of energy; even what appears to be solid matter is energy at its basic unit. In this way, your connection to all that is, to a source larger than yourself, is an energetic connection. You are energetically tapped in to the eternal wisdom that is held in the universe; you and the universe are of the same elements. In this way, there is spirituality because this connection is of a nonphysical nature. When you connect to all that is, you are tapping in to that part of you that is eternal and has the powerful healing potential of the source of energy of all that exists.

You also have the ability to move your awareness in the realm of bliss, or **Samadhi**. Meditation and **yoga nidra**, yogic sleep, are two vehicles that have the potential to take you to the experience of this state of awareness. This also is not religious belief. It is another state of awareness that is possible for you to experience when you deeply relax and just "be." In the peaceful experience that is called Samadhi, you experience your connection to all that is. And your body has time to restore and renew itself. You may also begin to realize the nature of life in ways that others cannot explain to you. When you open your eyes, after having meditated, you will often feel a sense of your wholeness. It's a comfortable feeling like pure love, and a stable contentment as though you've awakened from the perfect sleep and know and feel that all is well. When you've experienced this, it can be called a spiritual experience of recognizing your wholeness, your healing potential, and your connection to existence beyond just what you see, feel, taste, touch, and smell.

Ayurveda is founded on the belief in your connection to all that is. Ayurveda encourages you to believe that you have the ability to tap in to the healing power and wisdom that you seek. This wisdom is within you and all around you. The spiritual aspect of Ayurveda is that you are connected to the spirit, to the divinity that you seek. You are a co-creator in the healing energies that exist in the world.

Ayurveda Is Not a Fad

Though it's just starting to gain recognition in the West, Ayurveda has been practiced in India for more than 5,000 years. Ayurveda is not a quick fix nor a passing phase. Ayurveda offers guidance for how to reclaim your connection to natural foods and the natural rhythms of life in a way that will create health.

The recommendations of Ayurveda can be a natural extension of your life in a way that can be fun, enjoyable, and creative. These guidelines are not "have to's"; they can be "want to's" because they are ways for you to nourish and care for yourself and your family. Ayurveda teaches you how to live life and create health in a heart-centered and natural way.

CHAPTER 2

Why Ayurveda?

Would you like to flow through life with greater ease, contentment, mental clarity, and physical health? Would you like to feel a sense of empowerment and understanding when it comes to your overall well-being? Are you interested in preventing disease before it develops, knocks you down, or becomes life-threatening? If so, you will appreciate Ayurveda for its ancient wisdom and modern practicality. Ayurveda addresses the vitality of your entire being—body, mind, and life-force energy—for a life of balance, sustainable health, and longevity.

A Natural Way to Health and Joy

Just as trees, plants, and flowers are part of the natural world, so are you. The principles of the elements ether, air, fire, water, and earth are always at work inside of you and around you. As seasons change, as the time of day changes, and as years go by, your health depends on your ability to go with the natural flow of life. You and the natural world are in constant relationship. Ayurveda as a medical science is based upon this practical, real, and exquisite foundation.

Ayurvedic Recommendations Are Natural

The herbs, oils, and food suggested by Ayurvedic practitioners are made of all-natural ingredients. Unlike drugs that are prescribed as part of allopathic medicine, the regimens and herbs that make up the Ayurvedic lifestyle do not cause side effects. Using Ayurveda is a natural and safe way to improve your health and your relationship to the life you're living.

FACT

Ayurveda is a system of health for the entire family, not just for adults. And because there are simple ways of understanding the basic principles of Ayurveda, you can notice when you or your children are sliding out of balance. As you get to know yourself and your children, you can use Ayurvedic principles to sustain equilibrium and health.

As a natural way to health, Ayurveda recommends food, herbs, and oils that come from nature. Ayurveda also recognizes that your energy and thoughts toward the food you buy, prepare, and eat are as important as choosing the right ingredients. In other words, as you go shopping, as you cook, and as you eat, take time to appreciate the hard work and dedication of those who have made it possible for you to have this food. And if you grow your own herbs and food, you'll really notice your close relationship to what you are eating. Fill the food and the process of preparing it with your heartfelt care and love, and that energy will enhance the vital energy of the food. Also, get the freshest products you can find and afford.

Following Natural Cycles of Life

You may have noticed the many cycles of life. The moon has phases: new to full to new. The seasons cycle: spring, summer, fall, winter, spring. The sun rises, sets, and rises, and the days get shorter and longer as seasons cycle. There is a cycle of life as well, from childhood to young adulthood to the later years of life and then death. According to the tradition in India, where Ayurveda originates, birth-death-birth is also a cycle. After death, there is rebirth, and the cycle begins again. Just as there isn't a beginning and end to the way we see the sun rise and set and rise, there isn't a beginning or an end to life: life follows a cycle.

QUESTION

Do I have to believe in reincarnation if I'm interested in Ayurveda? Ayurveda is the science of life, so it focuses on the life you are living right now. The practices, advice, and recipes of Ayurveda deal with the here and now. So, you don't have to believe in life after death or reincarnation to benefit from an Ayurvedic lifestyle.

Ayurveda recognizes that as the seasons cycle, you are affected. And as you go through your cycle of life, your needs change. Ayurveda teaches about the qualities of the seasons of nature and of life, and it offers ways to stay in balance through these changes. There's a way to gently give in to the special attributes of each season while also making sure you stay in balance. This is how you'll remain healthy. For example, when the weather becomes cold and dry in winter, it affects you beyond a sense of physical discomfort. Winter is characterized as a vata time of year, and vata is associated with cold, dry, and mobile. In winter, the cold and dry air penetrates the skin, and it will affect bones, organs, muscles, and your body's biochemical processes if you don't add warmth and moisture to your body. For balancing the qualities of vata, particularly at this time of year, Ayurveda has natural, simple, and logical recommendations for lifestyle and diet to help warm you up and pacify the effects that winter could otherwise have on your physical and mental health.

Once you learn about your constitution and the qualities attributed to each season, you will be able to live in harmony with the natural rhythms of life. That way, you can remain healthy, comfortable, and immune to disease throughout the year.

Daily Cycles

Just as there is a seasonal cycle, there is a daily cycle. While temperature and the number of hours of sunlight will vary throughout the year and throughout the world, there is a natural daily cycle that remains the same. Instead of trying to plan your activities and routine in conflict with the daily cycle, it's best for your overall health if you work with the natural cycles of vata, pitta, and kapha as they occur each day.

▼ **2.1: THE DAILY DOSHA CLOCK**

Time of Day	Associated Dosha
6 A.M.–10 A.M.	kapha
10 A.M.–2 P.M.	pitta
2 P.M.–6 P.M.	vata
6 P.M.–10 P.M.	kapha
10 P.M.–2 A.M.	pitta
2 A.M.–6 A.M.	vata

The table of the daily cycle helps you understand when it's best to wake up (before kapha time), when to eat your biggest meal (lunchtime, pitta time), and what time to go to sleep (before pitta time) based on the qualities associated with each dosha.

A Whole System of Health

Ayurveda is a whole system of health. In other words, it recognizes the interconnectedness of your entire being: mind, body, and energy/spirit. When you exhibit symptoms of imbalance or disease, Ayurveda takes into consideration your mental, physical, and energetic/spiritual state. For example, if you have a headache, Ayurveda doesn't just look at what could be causing this from a physical perspective. Ayurveda is interested in your entire lifestyle and diet, even if the symptom seems to be clearly a headache. This is because all aspects of you are connected. Your body, mind, and energy system are connected. Disease that begins in the mind or energy body, if not addressed, spreads to the physical body. Disease in the physical body affects the mind and spirit. For this reason, Ayurveda as a whole system of health examines your lifestyle, your diet, your stress levels, your environment, and your relationships to create harmony and balance.

How to Achieve Perfect Health

The key to a healthy life, according to Ayurveda, is balance. Imbalance leads to disease. There are recognizable signs of early stages of imbalance that you can notice and correct before the imbalance creates further physical symptoms or advances to the stage of a life-threatening disease.

QUOTE

Health consists of a balanced state of the three humors (doshas), the seven tissues (dhatus), the three wastes (malas), and the gastric fire (agni), together with the clarity and balance of the senses, mind, and spirit. —Vasant Lad, BAMS, MASc.

When you visit with your Ayurvedic practitioner, she will want to get a clear picture of what you're managing in your life and how you are affected by it so she can make appropriate suggestions for adjustments in lifestyle, diet, and supplements. By making changes to your lifestyle and diet, you and your Ayurvedic practitioner will keep in mind the state of the doshas, dhatus, malas, and agni in you. And the goal is balance so you can live in harmony with the natural world and be immune to disease.

Ayurveda as Preventive Medicine

Ayurvedic practices are ways to take care of yourself so you don't get sick. As preventive medicine, Ayurveda is a way to maintain health. When you follow the wisdom of Ayurveda, you are maintaining your health on a daily basis; nourishing your mind, body, and spirit; and creating the conditions for

an easeful transition into the later years of your life. You do this by noticing early signs of imbalance and taking the natural methods prescribed by
Ayurveda to create equilibrium.

When Using Ayurveda as Complementary Medicine

Ayurveda is a system of health that stands on its own, as a way of life.
Because it is all-natural and supports all of you—mind, body, and spirit—it
can be used also as a complementary medicine. That means you can combine its practices with allopathic, or traditional, medicine.

ESSENTIAL

Ayurvedic herbs can interact with allopathic drugs. Always tell your
Ayurvedic practitioner and your doctor everything you are taking and
doing for your health to avoid adverse or unwanted side effects. You'll
need advice to be sure which Ayurvedic practices will be beneficial in
combination with the advice you receive from your primary care physician.

If you are seeing a Western medical doctor now, do not stop seeing her
if you want to begin to talk to an Ayurvedic practitioner. Continue with your
medical doctor, then meet with an Ayurvedic specialist or **Vaidya**, Ayurvedic
doctor, to see where she may be able to help. Always make sure that each
doctor you talk to is aware of everything you're doing for your health. Ease
into Ayurveda.

Complementary Therapies

In combination with your allopathic treatments, your Ayurvedic practitioner may recommend any of a variety of what Western medicine calls
complementary or alternative therapies. These therapies are called "complementary" because to traditional doctors, they are used as a complement
to their prescriptions—not instead of what they prescribe. They are called
"alternative" when they are used instead of allopathic medicine.

The following therapies are among those that your Ayurvedic practitioner may recommend. These therapies are all natural, have been used for thousands of years, and are used to restore your body by helping to circulate blood and lymph, support digestion, and boost immunity.

THERAPIES USED IN AYURVEDA

- **Aromatherapy:** using scents to pacify—or stimulate—the body and mind
- **Bodywork:** massaging herbalized oil over the entire body in rhythmic strokes
- **Marma Therapy:** applying pressure to specific points on the body to help energy flow
- **Mindfulness Practice:** becoming aware of what you are experiencing in each moment, which allows digestion, sleep, and other important physical and mental functions to occur naturally and easefully
- **Yoga, Meditation, and Pranayama:** cultivating mental equilibrium; promoting energy flow throughout the body; and enhancing physical strength, stamina, and health
- **Healing Modalities with Metals, Gemstones, and Colors:** using the energetic vibration of metals, gemstones, and colors to positively affect your energy system and overall health
- **Herbal Supplements:** ingesting natural, whole herbs and spices in powder, liquid, or capsule form to enhance the body's ability to detoxify, absorb nutrients, and regain equilibrium

Many people choose to follow Ayurveda because it's preventive and picks up where traditional medicine leaves off. It treats the person for all of who she is, and supports her in creating a sustainable lifestyle for a lifetime of perfect health. It can also be used as a support for the body and mind, when surgery or drugs are necessary.

Choosing Your Primary Care Doctor

If you are interested in natural ways of cultivating and maintaining health, you can find a doctor who practices **integrative medicine**. This means that he has been trained in allopathic medicine and has studied alternative therapies. This type of doctor would be very comfortable using a combination of allopathic treatments plus Ayurvedic recommendations to support your health in an ongoing way and during emergencies. An integrative doctor may not know a lot about Ayurveda, though she would recognize that true healing takes into consideration mind, body, and energy. Because of this, so she would support you seeing an Ayurvedic specialist for specific advice.

You can effectively integrate the modern and ancient systems of health. Many traditional doctors are interested in learning about complementary medicine. It's well known and widely accepted, now, that the mind and body are intimately connected and that the health of an individual affects and is affected by his day-to-day and moment-to-moment decisions and thoughts. By making choices for great health throughout your day, you support your immunity, your ability to deal with life's ups and downs, and your aging process. As you approach your decisions with intention about what to eat, whom to spend time with, and how to spend your energy, you will notice a change in your overall health. And this will decrease the amount of time you spend in a doctor's office.

Self-Empowerment for Health and Longevity

Ayurveda as "the science of life" gives you a lens through which you'll examine your life and your health. Once you understand the basics of Ayurveda, you'll have the potential for less confusion, less overwhelm, and less frustration when you are faced with early signs of imbalance, the precursor to disease. Early signs of imbalance include such familiar conditions as headache, constipation, sore throat, and irritability. When these types of early signs arise, Ayurveda tells you what immediate choices you can make that will support your immune system. You can turn to Ayurveda for guidance and natural recipes with herbs, teas, and spices that you can stock in your own kitchen.

It Just Makes Sense

Ayurveda makes sense. It demystifies the mystery of creating health. For those who don't gravitate toward science or aren't doctors, you may feel disconnected from any understanding of how to cultivate health. You may feel unable to understand what the body is, how it works, and how to work with it. Ayurveda doesn't require you to have an advanced biological or chemical understanding of the body. Instead, Ayurveda asks you to evaluate your health in terms of simple attributes. These are dry, oily, light, heavy, cold, hot, unctuous, rough, soft, hard, subtle, gross, mobile, static, clear, cloudy, slow, sharp, dense, and liquid. And as you read this book, you will see how logical and self-empowering it is to evaluate your health using these attributes.

ESSENTIAL

Remember, in Ayurveda, like increases like, and opposites balance. For example, if your vata dosha is aggravated, you will want to avoid cold, raw food and you'll want to limit sensory stimulation and movement. You will want to give yourself massages with warm oil, eat warm and moist food, and do yoga and pranayama practices that are grounding.

Once you understand the basics of Ayurveda, you can begin to incorporate the practices into your life. It can be a fun and nurturing experience to take care of yourself and your family in this way. Living healthily becomes a way of life and a way of love, not a chore or an unexplained mystery. And you can reduce your trips to the doctor by preventing seasonal allergies, flu, and other diseases and illnesses that take their toll on your body and your life.

Have Reference Materials and Support

What's great about Ayurveda is that you become a part of your own medical team. Your observations and participation in your own healing are as important as the Ayurvedic books you keep on hand and your visits with your Ayurvedic practitioners and your other doctors. You all work together in creating health for you and your family.

To support yourself, have books on hand that can remind you of what to look for as symptoms of early stages of disease and that offer great Ayurvedic recipes. See Appendix B for additional resources.

Notice How You Feel

Keep tabs on yourself and on your family. The sooner you notice signs of imbalance, the faster and easier it will be to correct them. The following are some questions to ask yourself to practice noticing how you feel.

- ❑ How do you feel physically throughout your body?
- ❑ How is your energy level throughout the day?
- ❑ How do you feel when you interact with others?
- ❑ What is your sleeping pattern: how long, light or heavy, dreams, nightmares?
- ❑ Are you feeling happiness and joy in your life?
- ❑ How do you feel at work?
- ❑ How many times per day do you have bowel movements?
- ❑ How many times a day do you urinate?
- ❑ Do you take time for relaxation?
- ❑ Are you completing important tasks?

As you read this book, you will become familiar with what your answers to those questions will tell you about your health. And you will learn and understand how to make adjustments in your lifestyle and diet when you notice imbalance. You will notice that by paying attention to your body and by nourishing and nurturing yourself you will create the conditions for your body to heal itself.

QUOTE

The blueprint for perfect health is inside you. It *is* you.
—Deepak Chopra, MD

When you talk to your Ayurvedic specialist, if you don't understand why he makes certain recommendations, then ask him why. Understand what you're doing for your health so you can continue to be an active participant in your wellness. With knowledge and understanding comes the ability to prevent disease from happening or from getting worse if it's already begun.

Keeping Your Family Healthy

Ayurveda isn't a medical system that you only turn to when someone gets sick. It's a way to create balance in your life, for thriving, longevity, and continued health. The wisdom of Ayurveda helps you determine the healthiest ways to cook your meals and spend your time, based on your constitution and the season. And because it's about your lifestyle, it's for the whole family. If you use Ayurveda for yourself and for your children, you will notice a more balanced household with less irritability and illness. When you aren't spending energy treating illness, you have time for the fun and educational things in life: family time, playdates, school, exercise, and other activities you'd choose for your family.

Cook with Your Children

Because the energy you put into your food enhances its nourishing properties, see if you can make it a fun, loving, and special experience to cook with your children. Allow them to be part of an aspect of preparing a meal, or see if it works for them to help by adding in spices. Lead them to put loving intentions into the spices before tossing them in. Explain to them what the foods are, how they are grown, and how they nourish the body and mind. Notice the colors, textures, and scents. Enjoy the preparation process together.

QUOTE

Meals which are lovingly prepared with a profound desire for the welfare of the eater always benefit the body and mind more than do meals which are commercially prepared, or which have been prepared by someone who is indifferent to or dislikes the proposed eater.
—Robert E. Svoboda, BAMS, in *The Hidden Secret of Ayurveda*

When the cooking experience becomes intentional, the nourishing and healing effects are heightened for the body and mind. Everything in the universe is made of energy; even matter when broken down to its smallest particle is energy. So the positive energy of your thoughts and intentions transfers into the food you prepare and serve.

ᴋids, Happy You

By using the wisdom of Ayurveda, you can keep colds and flu from entering the house and making the rounds, family member by family member. One of the best things to begin with is the practice of **abhyanga**, herbalized-oil massage. On top of having many important health benefits, abhyanga feels luxurious. The primary benefits of abhyanga are:

- Keeps the skin moisturized, preventing eczema and rash
- Supports the lymphatic system, which is how the body collects and removes pollutants
- Induces the feeling of being supported, balanced, and relaxed

Each of those benefits significantly supports the entire person: psychologically, physically, and energetically. In particular, oiling the skin has a direct effect on the lymphatic system, which is your body's way of capturing and removing the pollutants that can lead to allergies, colds, and flu. The oil penetrates into the deeper tissues, keeping them lubricated and able to support the various functions of the body, including the elimination of waste.

How and When to Do Abhyanga

Do abhyanga before entering the bath or shower in the morning. It's especially soothing to warm the oil first by running the bottle under warm water. Then, as you massage the oil into your skin (or your child's), massage in long strokes along the limbs, and massage in a circular motion over the joints. Be sure to massage the entire body, in loving strokes. This includes massaging oil into the scalp. Once your children are old enough, they can do abhyanga without your help. Learning to self-nuture is a wonderful skill for them to take into adulthood. If your child is predominantly vata or has a vata imbalance, it will help to give her a soothing foot massage with oil before she goes to bed.

Dynamic Approach to Overall Well-Being

Ayurveda is a dynamic approach to overall well-being because you and the seasons are constantly changing. As you change and as seasons change, your needs will change. The beauty of Ayurveda is that the advice it offers will feel natural to you. For example, in the summertime, especially if you are someone who has a good amount of pitta (the fire element), Ayurveda recommends cooling activities for the body, such as swimming (during the cooler hours of the day). As you and the seasons cycle and change, Ayurveda suggests modifications to your diet and activities to help keep you in balance.

The Benefits of Allowing Instead of Repressing

Because of the various to-do's in life and because of a variety of other reasons, you may find yourself repressing emotions and/or repressing certain bodily functions. In other words, what if you have a really busy week at work? You might not only repress feelings that you have so that you can get through the workweek, but you also might repress urges to go to the bathroom because you are just too busy. Repressing is unhealthy for the mind and body. When it comes to elimination, make time for elimination first thing in the morning. And listen to your body when it's ready to eliminate because that's its way of clearing the waste out of your body to keep you healthy.

ESSENTIAL

Allergies can be caused by repressed emotions. When you repress emotions, you create a vata imbalance. When vata is out of balance it affects agni, your digestive fire and your autoimmunity. If your autoimmune system is not acting and reacting properly, you could experience reactions to common allergens such as pollen and dust.

When emotions come up, give them space. If you're at work when emotions want to break through and you can't take a break, make time when you get home to allow the emotions. Feel them fully; breathe deeply in and out several times until the emotions eventually dissipate. You can think of the metaphor of riding waves. Be the surfer, who rides them without getting swept away by them. It could take some time for the sensations of the emotion to rise up and then float away. When you allow yourself to feel the emotions, they can pass through you. If you repress them, you carry them within the very cells of your body.

You may be repressing emotions for any number of reasons, so talking to a therapist, friends, and your doctors and healers about what you are experiencing is important. In addition, all aspects of your life contribute to how you will experience the emotions. What you eat, if you exercise, how well you sleep, and more contribute to your reactions to life and to your own emotions when they come up. Ayurveda is dynamic because your emotions and state of mind will shift, and Ayurveda can be there to support you with guidance for what to do when you experience different states of mind.

Find Time and Ways for Relaxation

In this fast-paced world, you may often feel stressed out and overwhelmed. When you become stressed out and overwhelmed, your body kicks in to fight-or-flight response. Your heart beats faster, your breath becomes shallow, and you may become tense. The body is not meant to stay in fight-or-flight mode. Fight-or-flight is meant for emergencies. The body needs periods in the relaxation response during which it will perform its normal functions. Your mind needs periods of rest, too, which you can give it through meditation, breathing exercises, yoga, and visualizations. And your energy body needs rejuvenation time: taking walks outside is a great way to restore your energy body.

QUOTE

In Ayurveda, a level of total, deep relaxation is the most important precondition for curing any disorder. —Deepak Chopra, MD, in *Quantum Healing*

The more relaxation time you can bring to your body, mind, and spirit, the more you will be able to make clear decisions in your life, enjoy physical health, and age well. Ayurveda gives you practical, simple, and effective ways to enhance your quality of life, which you will learn in the following chapters. And don't be surprised—though this will require some lifestyle and dietary changes as you adopt an Ayurvedic lifestyle, you could actually enjoy yourself! It's a nourishing, supportive, natural, and comprehensive science of life and longevity.

CHAPTER 3

Ayurveda and Yoga

Both yoga and Ayurveda originate in the ancient traditions of India, and they complement each other to support a healthy, easeful, and long life. Rishis realized Ayurveda as the answer to deep questions about how to nourish and heal the body, and they realized yoga as the way to understand the business of the mind. Practicing Ayurveda enhances the benefits of yoga, and yoga is a special part of your Ayurvedic lifestyle.

Why Practice Yoga?

The images of yogis twisting and bending their bodies into various shapes may lead you to imagine that yoga is a practice exclusively for the body. It's true that the physical postures of yoga are intended to release toxins from the body, create space, and lead to other physical benefits. It's also true that **hatha yoga**, the physical practice of yoga, illuminates the nature of the mind.

To understand the mind, you have to practice observing it. As you practice hatha yoga, you are able to watch your mind and watch what thoughts arise as you flow from posture to posture. Can you keep your mind steady and present, or does it wander and become restless? Can you return your attention to the breath and become present simply to the experience, without judging it? During your hatha yoga practice, observe that the mind likes to travel.

ESSENTIAL

During your hatha yoga practice, when your mind wanders, bring it back to the moment by noticing what parts of your body are touching the earth. Feel the support of the earth, then follow the breath. In hatha yoga, your breath supports your postures. You'll learn to coordinate your movements with your inhalation and exhalation for safety, ease, and stamina.

Hatha yoga is also a practice to prepare the body for meditation, stillness. Just as you can watch the activity of the mind during hatha yoga, you can watch the mind during meditation. **Meditation** is the practice of observing the mind and allowing thoughts to float by.

By first moving the body in hatha yoga, you will have an easier time sitting in stillness. From stillness, you observe the nature of the mind. You watch thoughts go by, without getting attached to them or continuing to follow where they lead. Every time you notice you have a thought, just bring your awareness back to your breath. Notice you are breathing, and watch the inhale and exhale. Notice the pause at the end of the inhale and the end of the exhale. As thoughts arise, gently bring your attention back to the breath.

The mind is restless. It plans. It thinks. It worries. There's a time and place for those functions of the mind. It's wonderful that the mind can be so adept and supportive of work and productivity. It's also important for you to learn how to create conditions so that the mind will rest, especially if it starts to spin in a stressful situation. Once you understand the nature of the mind, you are on your way to understanding how yoga and meditation are tools for the reduction of stress. Understanding this concept will support your Ayurvedic lifestyle. If you practice both Ayurveda and yoga, they support and enhance each other's effects, taking you toward deeper health of body, mind, and spirit.

How Yoga Reduces Mental Stress

Would you like better coping skills in the face of life's ups and downs? Would you like relief from spirals of depressive thoughts and anxiety? Would you like to know how to let go of anger and resentment? Yoga is here with the tools to help you.

Yoga teaches that in order to reduce the stress you feel, you must understand the nature of the mind. In your life, you will find yourself in situations that could lead you to feel stressed out, depressed, hopeless, alone, fearful, and anxious. You cannot control all the situations and outcomes in your life. Yoga teaches that you can learn practices designed to help you more effectively manage the stress you feel as a result of what happens beyond your control. When you understand the nature of the mind, you can change your experience of life and experience it with more joy, playfulness, and ease.

FACT

"Sthira Sukham Asanam" is one of the sutras, or threads of wisdom, in the ancient text *Yoga Sutras* by Patanjali. The translation of this sutra is "steady, sweet/comfortable posture." It means make your postures steady and comfortable. Do this with yoga postures on the mat and with postures you hold (physical, mental, and spiritual) throughout your life. This is yoga.

The *Yoga Sutras* were written by Patanjali to explain the science and philosophy of yoga. He didn't invent the study of yoga, but he is credited with writing it down in the poetic form that we have today. Each sutra is as short as one phrase or a few sentences, and they are threads of wisdom for you to contemplate as you move along your yogic journey toward understanding the nature of the mind. Here are the basic premises to understanding the nature of the mind, which is foundational to your peace of mind and your practice of Ayurveda, the science of life.

- You are not your thoughts; you are the one who can observe your thoughts.
- The mind is active—thinking, planning, judging, hoping, fearing, desiring, avoiding.
- When the mind is actively fearful, anxious, stressed, etc., that is not your true nature.
- Your true nature is Purusha, pure awareness.
- In order to experience pure awareness, you must learn to observe and calm the mind.
- Once the mind is calm, you experience peace, not stress, in your life.

Yoga and meditation are tools for learning to develop what is often called "witness consciousness," which is a way of saying that you are the witness to what is going on in your life. You are witnessing your thoughts, your reactions, and your emotions. You are not identifying yourself with them, as though you are them, nor are you getting caught up in them. You begin to recognize that your anger, your resentment, your guilt, your insecurity, etc., are not your natural state of mind. You, at your core, are at peace and equilibrium. Yoga and meditation teach you how to get in touch with that core and live from that place more often.

The Yoga Sutras

The *Yoga Sutras* were written in Sanskrit thousands of years ago (estimated dates range from 5,000 B.C. to A.D. 300), and now several translations and editions are available in English. Many editions exist that contain contextualization for each of the sutras, in addition to the literal translations. Because the sutras come from the ancient culture of India, you may find it helpful to read what the experts say about each sutra in the expositions printed next to the literal translation.

The second sutra is considered to be the foundational sutra, the entire purpose of yoga. It is "yogas citta vritti nirodhaha." In short, it means, "yoga is learning to live from the place of witness consciousness." Another way it's translated is "yoga is learning to restrain the modifications of the mind." In order to understand that sutra, you must understand the nature of the mind.

Why are there many translations of the same sutras?
Languages and cultures are constructed differently, and exact word-for-word translations do not always carry the meaning that's expressed in the original tongue. Translation is an art form, in which the translator aims to convey both literal and cultural meanings. Translations of the sutras use different English words, trying to help give a nuanced sense of the original Sanskrit.

The Nature of the Mind

The nature of the mind as described in this way is a new concept to many in the modern Western world. Before being able to restrain the modifications of the mind, you have to understand what the modifications of the mind are. This concept can be experienced in the following way.

Pause for a few moments, and see if you can watch your thoughts. Notice that you have the ability to watch thoughts that pass through your mind. Notice that your thoughts are fleeting or changing constantly. Recognize that you have the ability to view your life from a place of awareness that watches those passing thoughts and watches all you do and experience. You are both living your life and able to observe it.

When your mind has a thought, can you notice that you don't have to be thinking that thought? For example, if you are thinking about an apple, do you notice you can change that thought so you are now thinking about a lunch box? If you are thinking about what time to pick up your child from school, you could change that thought and think about mailing a birthday card to your friend. Your thoughts can change from moment to moment.

Sometimes you change the thoughts with your will, other times each thought comes and goes on its own. That is an essential component of the nature of the mind, that thoughts will come and go. You can watch them. You are connected to your mind, and you are not your mind. You witness it.

FACT

> If you are angry, you can separate from the anger to notice you are angry. If you are excited, you can notice you are excited. You as the witness can separate from the energy of the anger or excitement and watch it. That part of you, the witness, can observe with equilibrium the workings of the mind.

Once you understand that you can stand in the place of witness to your mind's activity, then you can understand the modifications—the stories—are what the mind designs. If, on the other hand, you identify with the movements of the mind as always true, you can lose touch with the present moment, reality, and balance. It's common to do this: the mind gets triggered and has patterns. That's why yoga is a practice. Life is constantly changing and you are confronted with new people and situations that can be challenging. Yoga helps you remember to connect to your witness consciousness, and it helps you start to do it as second nature.

The Modifications of the Mind

Sometimes the modifications of the mind are also called the "stories" of the mind. What do modifications of the mind look like? What are the "stories" that this concept refers to? It's not referring to the stories you tell others that you recognize as stories, like short stories, plays, or movies. The modifications of the mind are most noticeable when you have trouble seeing the truth or reality because your mind is caught up in a story, an assumption, or a guess that you construct about a situation or experience. Here's a scenario:

It's Pat's birthday, and last week her friend Julie said she'd meet Pat for a birthday lunch at Viva La Pizza, at 12:30. They confirm the date, time, and place a couple of days before Pat's birthday. On her birthday, Pat arrives at Viva La Pizza at 12:30 sharp. She doesn't see Julie anywhere.

Pat asks for a table for two and gets a lovely table by the window. She looks at the menu for a few moments, and then looks at her watch and sees it's 12:40. She feels some energy rise in her (a sensation, an uncomfortable feeling), and she starts to get concerned about Julie. It's 12:40. "Did Julie forget? Did she go to the wrong place? Is she okay? Maybe she got into a car accident." And Pat starts to worry that Julie got in an accident. Then Pat picks up her cell phone and calls Julie. Julie doesn't answer. Then Pat starts worrying, "She must be in trouble. She always answers her phone." Now, it's 12:45 P.M. Pat's worried energy is stronger, and since it's her birthday she starts to feel hurt and angry, imagining that maybe Julie didn't get in an accident. Maybe Julie has forgotten their date. Two more minutes pass, and Julie arrives. "I'm so sorry I'm late! I went to pick up a special birthday cake for you, and the line was really long. I was going to surprise you. Since I'm late I want you to know, I just handed it to the chef of this restaurant, and he'll bring it out after we eat pizza. I'm so sorry I'm late. Happy birthday."

In this scenario, the modifications of the mind are the "stories" Pat made up while waiting for Julie. The story begins when Pat spends time worrying if Julie got in an accident, and then Pat imagines her friend forgot her birthday. These are the stories, the modifications of the mind. The mind is modifying, or adding to, the reality. The reality in Pat's situation, while waiting for her friend, is simply that Julie is late. That's the reality. What her mind does, in response to the rising energy inside of her, is make up stories that cause her to suffer and feel stress—worrying that Julie got in an accident or imagining that Julie forgot the occasion altogether. The reason Julie was running late was nothing to worry about. She was trying to get a birthday cake, a pleasant surprise for Pat. That was the reality that Pat didn't know.

ESSENTIAL

The mind is a wonderful tool that can notice patterns and create organization. The mind is necessary for making plans, creating structure, and learning how to maintain safe conditions in the home. Learning witness consciousness doesn't mean disregarding the mind. It means being able to notice the mind's activity and deciding when to give it time to rest.

The example of Pat and Julie meeting for lunch illustrates how, by following the mind's stories once they start, you can cause yourself more suffering than if you stay in pure awareness, or witness consciousness. How would the scenario look different if Pat practiced being in witness consciousness rather than following the modifications of the mind? What is the alternative that the yogic and meditation practices offer?

Recognizing Rising Energy and Sensation

Before you begin to label something you experience as anger or frustration, see if you first just notice it as energy rising, or sensation rising. First, just notice the energy rise, and do not get caught in the mind as it starts to spin into a long tirade (e.g., "I'm so angry that my neighbor drove into my rosebushes again, he's so inconsiderate all the time, last week he . . ."). If you notice that happening, pause and focus on the energy that you are feeling. Pay close attention to the sensations. Note the location and quality of the sensations, e.g., tight, hot, gripping, clenched, dull, sharp, etc. In experiencing your emotions this way, you notice you'll feel the energy, you'll bring your awareness to it, and you won't fan the flames of your emotions by thinking more thoughts that cause more angst for you. Breathe through the sensations, focus on breathing in and out. Soon, the strength of your discomfort will dissipate and fade. And soon, the heated emotion (or energy) around what first arose will calm down. And you can then be in the situation with a level head.

For example, imagine you are at work and you have a deadline for a report in two hours. You feel energy around the approaching deadline. This energy could be something you'd also call anxiety or worry. As you focus on the report, all of a sudden your computer completely freezes. You cannot unfreeze it, and now you really get concerned. With this force of urgency, you call the technical help office in your building to let them know your computer has frozen. They tell you that the computers are down and they are doing what they can to fix them. They say it might take a half hour. You put the phone down, and then you get very angry. You get angry that you have to write this report, and then you think, "I wish I didn't have to be in the office on such a sunny day. And why can't these people fix the computers faster? I have a report due soon, what am I supposed to do? When will they get a better computer system for us, so this doesn't happen? The computers here are so out of date. This place doesn't appreciate me or the work I do here. I really don't like my job. I don't like working here."

What happens here is that you have a deadline, and you already have energy rising around that deadline. Then, when the computer freezes, you feel more energy rise and something else causes you to begin to follow the thoughts and spin in a negative direction. The spin in this scenario is that you start thinking that you wish you didn't have to be indoors, and then you go into a story about your employer not appreciating you and that you don't like your job. This story that you spin might cause you to dislike your job in the moment and construct a belief that your company does not value you, all based on the fact that you have a deadline and the computers are down.

FACT

Going outside if you are feeling tension is a great way to shift your energy. If you're cooped up inside, once you go outside you can connect to the spaciousness and beauty of nature. While you're out there, appreciate the moment, the trees you might see, and the fresh air. Cultivating gratitude is an antidote to stress.

Of course, the reality could be that you don't like your job, after all. Or, it could be that you do like your job, and sometimes the deadlines or the fact that computers will falter can cause you some stress. Either way, whether you do like your job or you don't, whether they do value you or not, is something that's better to think about from a more levelheaded place so you can really decide if you do or do not like working there. One deadline and a computer freeze might not be the best reasons for not liking your job.

Yoga for Levelheadedness

What yoga offers is the practice of cultivating levelheadedness by not attaching to the waves of thoughts. There is a way of stepping back and watching the energy rise, then allowing yourself to return to a place that is levelheaded. You do this by not attaching to the thought waves, not adding energy to the tides. This benefits you in the short and long run. To do this, in the aforementioned situation, you would notice the energy that you feel because of your deadline. You would notice the extra heat and energy are there. Just notice. Then, when the computer freezes and you learn it won't be up and running right away, you notice your energy rise. You notice it. And you watch the thoughts that come up. You notice the feelings and thoughts that come up about your workplace, and these are thoughts to look at again later once the energy has calmed down. Rather than continuing the path along the story you're creating now, that your workplace doesn't value you, that they'll never get new computers, and that you need to quit, just allow those thoughts to be there, and watch them without adding fire to them.

Watch and breathe. Take a nice, deep inhale and long exhale. Do this several times as you watch the energy rise and fall. Trust that everything will be okay. Keep watching the breath. Eventually, this energy you feel will pass if you don't keep feeding the fire with stories about how terrible computers are and that you want to quit. Nor is it better to repress the feelings and pretend they aren't there. That will make you tense, and the stored repressed emotions will stay in you, leading to imbalance and disease. So, just watch the thoughts, watch the energy, and breathe. Breathe. Every thought, every emotion is fleeting. This will pass. Breathe through it. Inhale and imagine you are inhaling calm energy; exhale the frustration and toxicity.

QUESTION

How do I breathe through difficult emotions?
When you feel stressed or anxious, it's likely that your breathing will become shallow and rapid. Gently begin to expand the belly as you inhale, creating space for more air to come in. Pull the belly button toward the spine on the exhale. Deepening the breath this way gently and patiently tells your body and mind it's okay to relax.

If you focus on breathing, soon the anxious energy will fade. And you will become calmer around the situation. Once you become calmer, you can think of what to do next. You could decide to take a walk for a half hour, and later you can make time to think about the difficult situations you are facing. You can think about that from a levelheaded place, not in the heat of the moment.

When you connect to that place of levelheadedness, you are connecting to your true nature. Your calm, centered, and balanced self is your true nature. There, you connect to wisdom beyond your emotions and frustration. You can create more ease, health, and happiness in your life if you make decisions from that place, your core and center.

Yoga's Holistic Model: The Koshas

The word yoga means "union." Yoga as union means that the goal of your practice is to experience the union of your consciousness and the universal wisdom of all that is. The physical practice of yoga opens you up to the experience of your true nature as a physical, mental, and energetic being.

Yogic philosophy describes the different aspects of your being as five different **koshas**, or sheaths. One way to visualize this is to imagine your physical body at the center of a bull's-eye configuration. Surrounding your physical body are energetic concentric circles, called sheaths. The innermost sheath is your physical body, and it is the densest. The outermost sheath is the bliss body, and it's the subtlest. See Table 3.1 for a list of the five koshas in order of densest to subtlest.

▼ 3.1: THE FIVE KOSHAS IN ENGLISH AND SANSKRIT

English	Sanskrit
Physical, or Food, Sheath	Annamaya
Breath/Energy Sheath	Pranamaya
Mental Sheath	Manomaya
Wisdom Sheath	Vijnanomaya
Bliss Sheath	Anandamaya

Your Physical Body

The sheaths are also referred to as bodies. It's just the terminology. It doesn't matter which term you use. The physical body refers to your physical form: your bones, muscles, organs, tissues, etc. This body includes the material aspects of you that survive and thrive on food, drink, and sleep.

When you see and touch the physical body, it feels solid. Yoga says the idea of the "solid" physical body is illusion. Science confirms it's an illusion. The basic unit of matter is an atom, which is energy. So your experience of solid form is illusion. The body is always changing at the cellular level. The very structure of physical matter is not solid; it's energy.

In Sanskrit the physical body is also called the **annamaya kosha**. The root *anna* means "food," and *maya* means "illusion." Although they are called illusions, the sheaths are a real part of your experience. They are veils through which you experience life. Ayurveda teaches you to understand what these veils are and to then work to become balanced in body, mind, and spirit for your overall health.

Your Breath Body

Your energy body, also called the breath body, is the **pranamaya kosha**, in Sanskrit. *Prana*, called ***chi*** in Chinese medicine, is the life-force energy that flows through the body. When you practice breath control exercises, **pranayama**, you control your breath and the flow of life-force energy.

Your Mental Body

Your mind and its myriad functions exist as the mental body. This is the aspect of you that experiences emotions, thought patterns, judgments, etc. This sheath is called the **manomaya kosha**, in Sanskrit.

The mental body is a place where perhaps you put most of your awareness. If so, you may not be making enough time to listen to the needs of the body and mind. Because of our expanding technology, you may find that when you aren't at work or doing your have-to's, your energy is focused on communication through the Internet and text messaging more than listening to what your own body and mind are asking for. The constant flow of short and prolific messages, abbreviated words, and rapid communication has people in the mental space of typing, reading, thinking, and responding in fast, exciting, and evolving ways. In this case, the benefit of the mental body is clear: the power of the thinking mind is able to advance technology and adapt to changing ways, connecting the people of the world in faster and more efficient ways. To balance this, take time for your body. And take time for some mental relaxation.

ESSENTIAL

You are an integrated being. Your mind and body communicate and respond to each other. When your mind feels stress, your body becomes tense, your breath shallow. When your mind is in a spin (of worry, anger, etc.), bring your attention to the body with a relaxing meditation or pranayama. As you relax the body, you will calm the mind.

Yoga and Ayurveda are in demand now because of a growing need to create a balance to our new speed, expansion, and rapid lifestyle. Yoga and Ayurveda do not ask you to stop your life as you know it. Yoga and Ayurveda offer tools to create health in this modern lifestyle.

Your Wisdom Body

Your wisdom body is the part of you that is a combination of what you've studied and how you've integrated it with your intuitive knowing. This sheath is called the **vijnanomaya kosha**. When you act from this place, you are trusting in the power of your intuition and connection to the wisdom of all that is. Making choices from here you are acting both with your acquired knowledge and with faith or trust in your inner knowing.

Your Bliss Body

You experience your bliss body when you are no longer experiencing life through your senses. You are in a deep meditative state, and you feel one with pure awareness. It is a place of feeling free, safe, connected, and peaceful. This is the **anandamaya kosha**; *ananda* means "bliss." Two ways to experience this are in meditation and in yoga nidra (yogic sleep). It's a state that is often described as being between sleep and wakefulness.

Yoga and Ayurveda: Sister Sciences

You can practice yoga without Ayurveda, and you can practice Ayurveda without understanding yoga. You will still receive benefits. You may also notice if you start practicing yoga that you will become interested in more ways to support your health in a complementary way, and Ayurveda will have answers for you. The same is true that if you start practicing Ayurveda, you may start having questions about your life and health that yoga may be able to answer because they stem from the same philosophy and support different aspects of your life and being. In this way, yoga and Ayurveda are considered sister sciences. They complement each other, flow together, and support you together.

What Yoga Can Do for Balance

In Ayurveda, to increase your health you will create balance, stabilize the flow of life-force energy (prana), and keep the digestive fire healthy. You don't have to imagine Ayurveda is asking you to cut out foods you love, while also asking you to accomplish the seemingly impossible task of cramming more lifestyle changes into your already packed schedule. Whether you are concerned about taking on a new practice because you feel too tired, too lazy, too overwhelmed, too overscheduled, too unhealthy, or too bored—if you are ready for better health, a radiant glow throughout your life, and peace of mind, it's time to create balance in your life. As part of your lifestyle, yoga can help.

HOW YOGA IS BALANCING

- Physical postures of yoga move your entire physical body, not just one part or side of you.
- The breathwork that accompanies the postures sends energy to every part of the body, including the brain.
- Yoga is much more than a physical practice; there are eight limbs to yoga that address the various aspects of your life.

Yoga is much more than physical postures. The physical postures are called **asanas**, and that is just one of the eight limbs of yoga.

Limb	Meaning	What It Is
Yama	Restraints	5 specific practices to help you navigate skillfully in the world
Niyama	Observances	5 specific practices to help you understand yourself in relationship to the world
Asana	Yoga posture	the word for "yoga posture"
Pranayama	Breath control	Breathing practices to help you control the flow of life force by controlling the breath
Pratyahara	Sense withdrawal	Practices to draw your awareness inward
Dharana	Focus	Practices to steady the mind
Dhyana	Absorption	Practices that unite you with the wisdom of the cosmos
Samadhi	Bliss	Feeling your existence as one with all that is

All of the eight limbs of yoga are practices to enrich your health and your quality of living. If you spend some time nurturing yourself by practicing each of these limbs, you will be supported in your body, mind, and spirit. One of the ways the eight limbs create balance is that you aren't just nurturing one aspect of your being. You are bringing health to your body, mind, and spirit. You are addressing all aspects of you, so there isn't one aspect that is overpoweringly strong and another that is depleted and neglected. You aren't just in your mind, or in your body, or in your spirit. You are pumping the muscles of each of those parts of you, keeping them vital and alive. And that creates balance, contentment, and the capacity for enjoying your life with health and vitality.

How Yoga and Ayurveda Work Together

The physical practice of yoga moves energy through the body. It creates space where there is tension or blockage, allowing the life-force energy that flows through you to reach all the parts of the body. Life-force energy is healing, rejuvenating, and balancing. As you practice yogic breathing, **pranayama**, and movement, you flood the body and mind with healing energy to support your sleep, your digestion, and your circulation.

As you move the body, you will notice that you enjoy feeling physically healthier. How can you support the physical body, in addition to the yoga postures? Ayurveda gives you the tools for how to nourish yourself: what foods to eat, when to eat, when to sleep, how long to sleep, how to notice if you're coming out of balance. Ayurveda tells you how to support the physical body, which includes having a physical practice of some activity and stretching each day that hatha yoga provides.

FACT

Ayurveda recommends that in your yoga practice, you do not strain. Ayurveda agrees with the yoga sutras, "make the posture steady and comfortable." It's best to move the body until you break a sweat, which is another way to release toxins. After you notice sweat all over, start winding down your physical practice, and end with stillness.

How to Begin a Hatha Yoga Practice

If you know you want better health and happiness, you must do something different to make a change. If you wish your health were different, you'll search for reliable and practical new choices for your health. Wishing or hoping things will change is an important step. Then turn those wishes or hopes into a strong intention to take steps in a positive direction. The hatha yoga practice is a wonderful way to start. You can start slowly and easily, even in as little as twenty minutes at a time.

What You'll Need to Start a Yoga Practice

There are a variety of yoga DVDs, CDs, and books available to help get you started. See Appendix B for additional resources. You can also find yoga studios or private instructors in your area. Many gyms have yoga classes, too. Not all yoga instructors and classes will be the same. You may want to ask friends or others for recommendations.

If you decide to go to a yoga studio, ask them to describe the kind of yoga they offer. Is it vigorous or gentle? Is it okay for beginners? Tell them your needs, and ask if that class is right for you. Also, ask if they provide mats and props, or if you should bring your own.

ESSENTIAL

As you look for a yoga studio, DVD, CD, or book as an introduction to yoga, take note that there are different types of yoga. Some are vigorous physically, others are gentle. Some are restorative, and some are practiced in rooms heated higher than 100 degrees. Some yoga classes are taught using many props, others use no props at all.

If you practice at home, the first thing you'll want to do is make sure you have space and the necessary props for your practice. You'll need enough space so you can lie down, stand up, and roll a little from side to side. The following props are good to have:

- A yoga mat
- A strap or tie
- Two yoga blocks
- A cushion or two
- A blanket

The yoga mat is to help you feel steady when you do the postures. It's not essential, though it does make practicing easier. It also keeps you off the hard ground when you lie down. You can buy a yoga strap or tie, or find a long belt around the house. The strap or tie is used as a way of reaching body parts you wouldn't be able to reach without the strap in your hands. Yoga blocks are useful as supports and so are cushions. Your yoga teacher can explain how to use the blocks and so can books and DVDs. A blanket is useful as a prop and also at the end of your practice to keep you warm. The last thing you will do after you practice yoga postures is to lie down and rest for several moments to allow the effects of your practice to integrate. In these final moments, you'll often experience a sound rest period. When you lie down for this last posture, **savasana**, or corpse pose, cover yourself with a blanket to keep warm. Your body temperature will likely drop when you relax so deeply.

Start Simply

You won't get faster results if you overexert yourself. Yoga isn't about overexertion. Yoga is about getting to know who you are, watching yourself as you do the postures. Are you trying to push too hard? Are you not pushing yourself at all? Are you listening to your body? Here are some general guidelines for beginning a yoga practice:

1. Follow your instincts when picking out a yoga studio, DVD, or CD—get what feels comfortable for you.
2. Keep your breath steady and smooth as you practice. Your breath is your support and your connection to life-force energy, prana.
3. Yoga is a practice, and you'll understand it more and more with time. Do not pressure yourself to have to look a certain way or feel something you don't feel. Practice being okay with where you are: that in itself is a key to yoga.
4. If you feel sharp pain, come out of the posture.
5. Every posture has contraindications, so talk to your doctor and health-care practitioners before starting a new practice.
6. Allow yourself to let go and let the experience be what it will be. Each time on the mat will likely feel different to you. It's new each time, just like each day is a new day.

The physical practice of yoga isn't meant to be serious, tense, and difficult. It's meant to be steady and sweet. It's meant to create space in the body and in the mind. As you begin your practice, just breathe. Take in one breath at a time. And smile.

Yoga for the Whole Family

Yoga is a practice that can be done by the whole family. The postures can be fun, funny, and joyful. The postures can also be deep, challenging, and fortifying. Everyone can learn ways to modify postures so that they are safe and comfortable. You can find guidelines for posture modifications for different ages and physical types. People of all ages will benefit. And it's fun to do with others.

Children, Teens, and Yoga

Many babies naturally put themselves into positions that are part of a hatha yoga sequence. Poses such as Happy Baby, Down Dog, Cobra, and Plank, which adults do in their classes, many children do on their own even before they learn to speak or walk.

QUESTION

Do I have to practice yoga every day to receive the benefits?
You don't have to practice every day, though regular practice, even ten minutes on days when you are short on time, will yield noticeable benefits. The more you practice, the more you will experience consistent and deep effects. If you have stressors in your life, your yoga mat is the place to practice letting it all go.

Yoga is safe for children, and as they get older yoga can support them through high school and adulthood. Because yoga helps calm the mind and create physical health, it's a wonderful constant in a person's life. Because throughout life, everyone is changing and experiencing change, the yoga mat is a place to find your center, no matter what age.

Partner Yoga

A fun way to practice yoga in the family is to try partner yoga poses. Partner yoga helps build connection between two people, and it's fun. When you are in a partner yoga posture, you and your partner are practicing communication. You'll ease into postures together, hold, and then help each other release the posture. You can communicate with your voices and also with the energy of the body.

A PARTNER YOGA POSE

1. Stand with your partner shoulder to shoulder, facing the same direction, holding hands, with your inside feet touching.
2. Each take a big step to the side with the outer foot, turning that foot out 90 degrees.

3. Keep a good, strong hold, and bend the outer leg, sending the knee in the direction of the middle toe. The outside arms lift to shoulder height and reach out in the same direction as the foot. Head turns to look over the outstretched hand.
4. Check in with your partner. Make adjustments for special needs and for comfort.
5. Hold for 3 to 4 breaths. Explore this pose with great support: experiment by sinking deeper into it.
6. When you are ready, tell each other, and gently release the pose by bringing yourself back to the starting position.
7. Thank your partner, and change positions. Repeat on the other side.

Partner yoga is an enjoyable way for you to practice asanas with others. When you practice partner yoga, it expands your practice in a new direction, and you learn to communicate with another person through vocal communication and physical energy. Also, for parents, it's a chance to connect and play with your children in a healthy, physical way.

CHAPTER 4

Visits with an Ayurvedic Practitioner or Consultant

Visits with an Ayurvedic practitioner help you feel empowered. During your visit, she will ask about a variety of aspects of your life, including the symptoms or ailments you are presenting. By answering her questions, you'll tell her how you are holding up psychologically, physically, and energetically so she can make natural and holistic suggestions for your overall healing. Her recommendations will help you understand what you need, and why, to deal with your present symptoms and get on the path to long-term health.

The Questionnaire

Before visiting your Ayurvedic specialist, you will fill out a questionnaire. The questionnaire will give your practitioner information about your health history and how you are feeling now. The questionnaire is likely different from what you experience with most Western doctors because it's designed to give a full picture of how you are living your life, not only focusing on disease or pain.

Topics Covered in the Questionnaire

Not all questionnaires from Ayurvedic practitioners will be the same, but they will generally cover the same topics. Here are some areas of your life the questionnaire will cover:

- Your family's health history
- Your present symptoms and their duration
- Any medications you might be taking
- Your eating, sleeping, and exercise habits
- What tastes you crave
- The frequency and qualities of your elimination (stool and urine)
- Your energy level

The specific questions will guide you toward painting a full picture of your lifestyle and habits. For example, regarding your sleeping habits, they will want to know what time you go to bed, what time you typically wake up, whether your sleep is heavy, if you have nightmares, and whether you wake up refreshed.

Something unique about the Ayurvedic questionnaire is that it will ask how you would describe your family life, social life, work life, and spiritual life. Your relationship to these components of your life can affect your health, and can also give your practitioner more information about your prakruti and vikruti.

What You Can Learn from the Questionnaire

There are no "right" or "wrong" answers to the questions. They are designed to help your practitioner gauge how you are and what kinds of changes could support your healing and continued health.

ESSENTIAL

When filling out the Ayurvedic questionnaire, do your best to answer the questions as truthfully as you can. It is suggested to answer the questions by looking at yourself through time, from childhood to present, and answer from what has been most consistent in your nature over time and, most especially, how it showed up in childhood.

The questionnaire is designed to help your practitioner understand various aspects of your life, and you, too, can learn a lot about yourself and your lifestyle as you fill it out. In this way, the questionnaire is a guide that helps you learn what to notice about yourself. It may present questions about your diet or lifestyle that you never thought to notice, and so now you can take the time to notice and your practitioner can help you make healthier choices.

Pulse Diagnosis

Your Ayurvedic specialist will be able to understand a lot about the health of your body by reading your pulse. Pulse diagnosis is a foundational, intricate, and unique aspect of Ayurveda. Modern Western doctors also use the pulse as a means for determining certain health factors, but Ayurveda uses it in a more detailed way to discover much more about what's going on with your body, mind, and energy flow.

Feeling and Listening to the Doshas

Your Ayurvedic practitioner will use your pulse to discover many things about your health, including how the doshas are showing up in you. The pulse diagnosis is the way your practitioner can really listen to what your body has to say and tune in to how your life-force is flowing.

Ayurveda contains extensive instruction and wisdom about the various aspects of health that a practitioner can determine from the pulse. It takes practice, study, and sensitivity to be able to interpret the numerous types of messages that the pulse contains. In keeping with its connection to nature, Ayurveda uses animals as metaphors for how the pulse moves. Vata in balance feels like the movement of a cobra, pitta in balance hops like a frog, and kapha in balance glides like a swan.

The Sanskrit literature contains a number of words that can be translated as pulse. The most commonly used word is nadi, which means a river of life expressed through the pulse. [Another] synonym is tantu, which means the string of a musical instrument through which one can listen to the music of feelings and emotions. Hence, pulse is also called tantu. —Dr. Vasant Lad

There are various parts of the body where you can have your pulse taken. Often the radial pulse, near the wrist, is a common place to read the pulse.

What Advanced Practitioners Can Determine

With study and practice, a well-trained, skilled, and sensitive practitioner can use pulse diagnosis to determine the condition of your doshas and much more. The pulse diagnosis is an important part of the visit between you and your practitioner. It helps support and add important information to the other components of her evaluation.

Your Physical Appearance and the Doshas

Your internal world and external appearance are connected. What's happening inside of you, mentally, energetically, and physically, will show in your physical appearance. When it comes to the doshas, the way the qualities of the elements are acting in you will cause certain signs in your physical appearance. Your Ayurvedic practitioner can notice qualities in your physical appearance that reflect qualities associated with vata, pitta, and kapha.

Vata

Signs of strong vata are dry and brittle nails and hair. A person of vata constitution will usually have small eyes. He will have a thin body frame, and skin that is dry and rough.

If you think about the qualities of vata—dry, rough, and cold—then it makes sense that the physical qualities associated with vata would be dry hair, nails, and skin. The qualities of air and space in the body make it thin, brittle, and dry.

Pitta

A person exhibiting pitta qualities will have penetrating eyes, usually green or gray. Her nails will be healthy and smooth. Her body's frame will be of moderate size, her skin oily and warm, and she'll easily perspire. Her hair could be red and go to gray early. She may have freckles, on her fair, red, or yellowish skin.

With the elements of pitta being of both fire and water, pitta's outward show is wet, hot, and sharp. And those qualities will show up in the hair, nails, skin, and other body parts.

Kapha

Kapha's eyes are large, round, and have thick eyelashes. The nails are thick and strong. A kapha's body type is large and round, and his skin is oily and pale. His hair could be thick and oily, and his teeth strong and white.

Kapha is a combination of earth and water, so thick, heavy, and wet qualities will show up outwardly. Coolness is also associated with kapha, so kapha's skin may be cool to the touch.

Tongue Diagnosis

The tongue is an important part of your digestive process. It helps move food around in your mouth so you can chew it, and it provides saliva to help break down food. The tongue is also an indicator of how well you are digesting and absorbing nutrients.

FACT

When you stick out your tongue, if you notice that it trembles or is shaky, that's a sign that you're experiencing fear and/or a fair amount of stress. Take a moment now, see if your tongue is shaky when you stick it out. If so, is it accurately reflecting that you feel fear or stress?

By looking at your tongue, your practitioner will be able to realize how your colon and small intestines are doing, as well as other parts of your body, including your heart, spine, lungs, and kidneys.

There are many more evaluations your practitioner will be able to make based on these and other aspects of your physical appearance. Ayurveda is a vast science, and your outward appearance can reveal so much about your internal state of being because you are a whole, interconnected being. What goes on for you internally will reflect externally.

Sitting Down for a Heart to Heart

Ayurveda puts great emphasis on your emotions, thoughts, and beliefs because they all influence your health. Love and kindness are healing. When you go in to visit with your Ayurvedic practitioner, you are entering a place where he will see you as a full being. He will not be looking at just your symptoms and their biological functions. He will be sitting with you, listening to you, talking to you, and wanting to assess how the various aspects of your life combine together and determine how you are feeling now. You can come to the meeting with the intention of openhearted and safe discussion, where you are being seen as a total and unique person.

Taking Your Time

As your Ayurvedic practitioner asks you questions, you can take a moment to think about the answer. Sometimes it might take you some time to think about an aspect of your life you haven't been noticing or thinking about. So, don't feel you have to say the first thing that comes to mind. Giving accurate information is more important than rushing.

ESSENTIAL

From an Ayurvedic perspective there are various ways to handle symptoms (like a headache or diarrhea) because you want to treat the underlying cause not suppress the symptom. By treating the underlying cause you create health in the body; by suppressing a symptom you can potentially create more disease or at the very least have the symptom return.

As you meet with your consultant, ask questions if there's something you don't understand. When you go home later to follow his advice, it will help if you understand why you are doing what you are doing. Your understanding and visualizations of the healing process really do support its efficacy. You are a key participant in your healing process, and your Ayurvedic practitioner provides his expertise and guidance to help you along the way.

New Topics on the Table

When you talk with your Ayurvedic practitioner, you may find yourself discussing topics that you aren't used to having on the table with doctors. The topics will include your elimination, your diet, your relationships, and your work life. These could feel like personal topics, and you may not be used to discussing them with your doctors.

ESSENTIAL

When talking to your practitioner, try to let go of any judgment you have about your health. If you have diarrhea, your tongue is coated with a white film, and/or your nails are brittle, allow all of that to be the truth, without judgment. Just notice how you are, and cultivate compassion for your body and all it's coping with.

There's good reason for why a variety of subjects will come up when you talk with your Ayurvedic specialist. Hearing about the various components of your life informs your practitioner about how the doshas are working in you and how your environment might be affecting you. From there, she can give sound advice about how to create balance, good digestion, and lasting health.

The Recommendations You Can Expect

When you visit with your Ayurvedic specialist, he'll ask about your lifestyle and diet before making recommendations for your health. Specifically, some of the topics he'll be most interested in discussing are your eating and sleeping habits, how well your digestion is functioning, and how you're dealing with stress. After your discussion, his pulse examination, and his observation of your physical attributes, your Ayurvedic specialist will make recommendations for you to incorporate into the foundational aspects of your life, such as sleeping, eating, and exercising.

Getting a Good Night's Sleep

A good night's sleep is important for your overall health, and you can allow nature's clock to help support your sleep. The hours of 6–10 P.M. naturally have the qualities of kapha. So if you can fall asleep by 10 P.M. the qualities pervasive in the outside world will help you drift into sleep. The hours from 10 P.M.–2 A.M. are characterized as pitta time, so if you aren't asleep before 10 P.M., your body and mind may be influenced by nature's fiery qualities, which will make it harder for you to fall asleep. Because it's pitta time from 10 P.M.–2 A.M., it is the time of night when your body would like to be digesting. If you're sleeping, it's a great time for your body to be able to focus on digesting everything you've taken in during the day while you are resting your senses.

If you have trouble falling asleep, your Ayurvedic specialist can make some recommendations for what to do to help you ease into sleep. One thing she may recommend is self-massage:

BEDTIME SELF-MASSAGE WITH WARM OIL

1. Heat sesasme oil for the vata and kapha body types and coconut oil for the pitta types until it's warm to the touch.
2. With slow, soothing strokes, massage your feet with the warm oil.
3. Wash your hands and cover your feet with socks so you don't stain your bedsheets with oil.
4. Massage warm oil along the brow line and at the crown of your head as you take deep, soothing breaths.

Along with self-massage, your specialist may recommend that you try certain herbs, tea, or warm milk before crawling into bed. What she recommends will depend on what she determines is causing you to be imbalanced and unable to fall asleep.

A Good Time to Wake Up

Nature supports your falling asleep and your waking up. Vata time is 2 A.M.–6 A.M., which is the time when people may find themselves naturally waking up even if they'd rather be sleeping. Waking up before 6 A.M. (or sunrise) is ideal because 6 A.M.–10 A.M. is associated with kapha. If you wait until after sunrise to wake up, you'll be struggling to wake up during nature's kapha time. You'll feel the qualities of that time of day, which are sluggish, heavy, and unmotivated as you start your day. If you wake up during vata time, you'll be assisted by those qualities that support the movement of mind and body.

Recommendations for Eating

Your Ayurvedic specialist will recommend whole foods you can gravitate toward and foods that would be better for you to avoid, based on how you are when she sees you. This will change a little bit when the seasons change and as the doshas in you become balanced and imbalanced based on various factors.

QUESTION

When's a good time to eat the biggest meal?
Because 10 A.M.–2 P.M. has pitta qualities, this is the best time to eat your biggest meal. You'll likely be hungry at this time and ready for good digestion because of the fiery qualities of pitta. This fiery time of day supports digestion.

In addition to certain foods, your specialist will likely recommend herbs, teas, oil, powders, and spices for you to add to or eliminate from your diet. All the recommendations are natural, and you can stock your kitchen with them so they are easily accessible when you're cooking and eating.

When cooking for an entire family, if you have a family of various constitutions, you can make recipes that are tridoshic—good for balancing all doshas.

Getting Exercise

Movement is very important for your body. It lubricates the joints, aids in digestion, keeps bones strong, helps the flow of fluids in the body, and can be used as an aid for balancing your doshas. Your specialist will take into consideration your constitution, your symptoms, your time of life, and the time of year when she recommends exercise for you. One thing for you to keep in mind is that like increases like and opposites balance. So, for example, if you are predominantly pitta, in your pitta stage of life, and it's summertime, you'll want to avoid vigorous exercise in the heat of the day because that will aggravate pitta in you.

Alternative Therapies

There are a number of alternative therapies that your Ayurvedic specialist may recommend to support your health. Some alternative therapies that support the Ayurvedic lifestyle are Ayurvedic bodywork (massage with warm, herbalized oil), marma balancing therapy (energy work), yoga, meditation, and aromatherapy.

An Ongoing Relationship with Your Specialist/Practitioner

For continued health and vitality, you can stay in consistent touch with your Ayurvedic specialist. As you experience change in your life, in your mental and physical state, and with age, you can make modifications in your diet and lifestyle. As seasons change, too, you will make some adjustments.

Sustaining Health by Supporting Yourself Daily

When you follow Ayurveda's wisdom as your primary model for healthy living, your focus is on maintaining strong immunity through your diet and lifestyle choices. Instead of waiting until you're sick to focus on taking care of yourself, you maintain your body, mind, and heart so that they can perform their functions to keep you healthy and happy.

ESSENTIAL

> To stay healthy, your body, mind, and heart will need to be able to digest all the experiences you have. As an integrated being you process food, thoughts, emotions, sensory input, and everything else you encounter. Ayurveda helps you do this with a variety of tools to support the functions of your mind, body, and spirit day by day.

For you, this may be a completely new way of thinking about health, and it might seem hard to imagine the real benefit of preventive care. If so, try to imagine that you are preventing illness the same way you prevent your car from breaking down. You get regular oil changes to prevent serious mechanical problems. You fill your car with gas before it becomes empty. You take care of your car to prevent breakdowns and to help it stay in great condition as it gets older. You can do the same thing for your health and your body. You can maintain your health to prevent breakdowns and the development of disease. As you maintain your health, you also age with more radiance and ease.

In Partnership with Your Practitioner

As you notice changes in your health, or if you have questions, keep in touch with your practitioner. She can continue to make recommendations as you and your life circumstances shift and change. You two will be working together in partnership for your sustained health. She can assess your needs for support, and then you will play an active role in your healing. To be able to help both you and your practitioner support your health, you can:

- Notice how your body feels, what your mood is like (and if/when it changes), how your sleep is, how your digestion is, and how your mind is working.
- Follow the recommendations from your practitioner, and be consistent.
- Trust your instincts if something isn't feeling supportive to you, and talk about it.
- Have positive, healing intentions around your body and heart, mind the food you prepare, and follow the advice of your specialist.
- Envision yourself whole, healed, vital, strong, and radiant.

The relationship between you and your Ayurvedic specialist is an important part of your healing. Make sure you are feeling comfortable with her and that you trust her. Your belief in her Ayurvedic recommendations is an important part of your healing, so if you don't trust her then find another specialist whom you can trust and believe in.

In addition to your specialist's advice and support, your health depends on your commitment to making healthy choices and your belief in your ability to be well. You really are the one who heals yourself, and your Ayurvedic practitioner guides you and supports you along the way.

CHAPTER 5

Naturally Beautiful Lifestyle

Have you ever been in awe of the beauty of the natural world? Have you ever realized there is beauty all around, and all you have to do is pause and notice? Nature is beautiful and alive. The fruits of the earth and the energy of the elements are at once pleasing to the senses and essential to life. The expansive possibility of space, the coolness of a summer breeze, the bright heat of fire, the nourishing flow of water, and the energetically rich soil have the qualities to support your health and well-being.

Align Yourself with Nature's Healing Potential

The natural world is full of the "medicine" your body needs. Food, spices, herbs, and the elements contain the ingredients and properties you need for health, radiance, and longevity. You may not be accustomed to thinking about how intimately you are connected to the natural world. You need space, air, fire, water, and the earth to sustain you, and you exchange life-force energy with all that is.

If you acclimate yourself to your inherent relationship to nature, you will enjoy greater health. To do this, take the time to cultivate a felt sense of your connection to the outdoors. Once you begin to feel it, you will understand it to be so. One simple way to begin to notice the healing effects of the natural world is to go outside more often. See if you feel the connection. Here are ways to incorporate outside time into your day, to lean into the healing power of the natural world:

- Before checking e-mails, making phone calls, or doing any work, in the morning take a walk or have a cup of tea outside, even if for just ten minutes.
- Throughout your workday, step outside for short breaks. Take nice, deep breaths. Gently stretch and shake out your limbs.
- Schedule and plan outside activities with your family.
- Take time before bed to go outside and notice the night sky. Breathe the fresh air, notice what's around you. Even if just for a few moments, allow yourself this connection to nature that will divide the energy of your busy day from your preparation for sleep.

ESSENTIAL

Nature is balance for you. If you're feeling tense, the outdoors can bring calm; if you're feeling sluggish, the outdoors can revitalize you. All you have to do is get out there, stand on the earth, breathe, and open to the shift that you need for balance.

Remember, if you are reluctant to take a break, it isn't just that it "feels good"—it really is necessary and good for you. It's a way to start taking care of yourself in just a few moments at a time throughout the day. You will begin to notice the effects, and you'll know from the experience that going outside is so important.

Natural Healing Power

If you begin to live your life with more enjoyment of what's natural in the activities you plan and in the foods you eat, you will start to gravitate toward a healthier and happier lifestyle. You don't have to give up your e-mail and Facebook time, your favorite TV shows once or twice per week, or your occasional unhealthy foods. Begin to cut back, though, and fill in the extra time in ways that you can connect with friends, animals, and nature.

FACT

A great activity that connects you to nature is starting a garden. You can even start with a simple herb garden. Or you could just grow one or two foods, such as lettuce and snap peas. You'll be reminding yourself and your family of where your food comes from and how miraculous and fun it is to watch it grow.

Ayurvedic specialists understand the healing potential in whole foods, herbs, and spices. Herbs will vary in potency, so it's important for you not to guess or experiment on your own. There is so much healing available to you in the natural world, and with the advice of a trained practitioner you can enjoy immunity and vitality, naturally.

Walking Meditation

A walking meditation is a wonderful way to attune yourself to the rhythm and wisdom of the natural world. Your walking meditation takes you into the present moment, where you can allow other thoughts to drift by. It creates space and time for you to appreciate and connect to nature, which is so important for your understanding of yourself and holistic, natural healing.

A WALKING MEDITATION

1. If it's cold outside wear enough layers to be warm. If it's hot out, be sure you can remove layers to be comfortable. Check the weather so you can enjoy your walk.
2. After stepping outside, take a nice deep breath and let out a long exhale. Do this a few times.
3. Set an intention for your walk. For example, "I'm taking a break now; there's no work for me to do on this walk. I can relax and be present to what is." Or, "I'm so grateful to live among such beauty, I'm going to spend some time appreciating it."
4. As you set out on your walk, intend to stop along the way or before you turn around to come back. Use those pauses to notice the world around you. In the summer, stop to notice the details on the flowers, and see if a butterfly stops by. If it's wintertime, admire the translucence of icicles. Touch, smell, listen, and watch the world around you.
5. As other thoughts come to mind, allow them to be there. Then, bring your awareness back to exploring what's around you.
6. As you walk, when you're not admiring the changing natural world around you, notice how it feels when each foot touches the ground. Notice your posture. Notice how it feels to bring energy into the leg muscles. Swing the arms as you walk, get the bodily fluids flowing and pumping. Enjoy the movement.
7. When you've completed your walk, spend a moment in gratitude for that time outdoors. Allow that moment to be your acknowledgment of the good you've just done for your health.

Going on a walking meditation is healthy for your body, mind, and spirit. The mind gets a break, the body gets movement, and your spirit connects to the thriving life-force energy that's all around. If you go with your children, partner, or friend, remind each other of the beauty that surrounds you: the way the sun is hitting the trees, the sound of a bird that you can't see. What can you notice and share?

Create Conditions for Balance Each Morning

Begin to connect to the rhythm of the natural world the moment you wake up. Ayurveda provides you with a nourishing paradigm for starting off your day. Can you imagine how your day might feel different if you were to take some time to smoothly transition from sleep to wakefulness first thing in the morning? Do you already smoothly transition from a sleeping state into the rest of your day, or do you hop out of bed and rush to get going? Or are you so lethargic that you can't get out of bed, and when you eventually do get out of bed your day starts off slowly and sluggishly so that you're running behind and feeling out of it? Ayurveda recommends a morning routine to help you start your day off from a good place.

Why Transition from Sleep to Morning Activity?

You may not know this, but the rhythms of the natural world support you in making a transition from your night of sleep to your morning of activity. If you don't take some time to transition, you're not listening to what your body and mind need. After being asleep for seven to nine hours (the ideal amount of time to sleep), your body and mind need a little space and care so they are ready for the big day ahead.

QUESTION

What if I'm a parent and don't have time for myself in the morning? If somehow you can get up twenty minutes earlier than the rest of the family to do at least some parts of the routine for yourself, that would be wonderful. And these routines are also helpful for children (in modified form, depending on their ages. Talk to your Ayurvedic specialist about it).

Ayurveda teaches a nurturing and balancing way to transition from your nighttime stillness to morning activity. By doing this you create a smooth transition from sleep to activity, integrating the benefits of your sleep and creating a good foundation. After your morning routine, you are ready to begin your day from a place of centered groundedness. The morning routine also supports the flow of bodily fluids (such as blood and lymph), builds immunity, creates mental stability, prepares the body for movement, and much more.

Everyone can end up feeling so busy nowadays, having not one moment to spare. In fact, it's because of that feeling that people have become distanced from nature and the needs of the mind and body. This disassociation from your needs and from nature's rhythm leads to imbalance and disease. Keeping up this daily nourishing morning routine is a good way to discipline yourself to take time for yourself. You'll feel real health benefits if you are consistent.

The Ayurvedic Morning Routine

There are specific components to the Ayurvedic morning routine, making sure you take care of the mind, body, and the sense organs. See Table 5.1 for the components and their benefits.

▼ 5.1: AYURVEDIC MORNING ROUTINE

The Practice	The Benefit
Use a tongue scraper	clears the undigested waste from your mouth
Use a neti pot	clears the nasal passages
Use nasal oil	keeps the nasal passages moist and creates less inviting conditions for bacteria or allergens to stick
Oil in the ears	keeps the ears healthy
Spray rosewater in eyes	moistens the eyes and relieves burning or itching
Massage your entire body with oil	lubricates the skin, joints, and organs; stimulates lymph and blood flow for immunity; grounds the mind and body
Drink a glass of warm water	supports morning elimination of waste
Joint warm-ups and yoga	prepares the body for movement
Take a walk outside	connects you to nature, gives your lungs fresh air, gets the body going
Pranayama, a breathing practice	helps center you and prepare you for the day

During sleep, your body has time to restore. It als[...]
functions, including digestion. When you wake up, if [...]
the morning routine, you clean out your sense orga[...]
nation of toxins after your body has performed dig[...]
the night. You'll be starting your day clean, fresh, an[...]
balance.

HOW TO DO THE MORNING ROUTINE

1. **Scraping the Tongue.** This will clear the **ama**, undigested substances, off your tongue. Use a metal tongue scraper, and carefully swipe it across the tongue until what you scrape off is clear. In between swipes, rinse the scraper off under warm water.

2. **Neti Pot and Nasal Oil.** This part of your routine will keep the nasal passages clean and moist, which will keep bacteria and other foreign particles from settling into your body's system. To do this, buy a ceramic neti pot, and follow the instructions that are included on the box or inside the box. You will need warm water and noniodized sea salt. After using the neti pot, carefully tilt your head from side to side over the sink so all the water comes out. Then, use nasya (or sesame) oil. To do this, lean your head back, and drip a few drops of oil into your right nostril. Keep your head back for about thirty seconds and massage the oil into the nose. It's okay if some slides down your throat. Bring your head to a neutral position for a moment. Then, tilt your head back and repeat the steps on the other side by dropping oil into your left nostril. Once on each side, each morning.

3. **Oil in the Ears.** Place oil on your fingers and gently and carefully rub the inside and the outside of each ear. Be sure to massage the ear lobe, too.

4. **Rosewater Spray in Your Eyes.** This keeps your eyes moist and clear. It's especially helpful during allergy season.

5. **Self-Massage with Oil.** If you are primarily vata or kapha, use warm sesame oil. If you want to pacify pitta, use coconut oil. Begin your self-massage by massaging your arms. Use long, steady strokes on the long bones, and use a circular motion to massage oil into the joints. Do the same for your legs. Continue to massage every part of your body, giving it loving,

soothing attention. The oil will sink into the skin and lubricate deep tissues. It will create healing on deep levels, beneath the skin. You can also oil your head. The oil will come out of your hair if you use shampoo. You can shower after you give yourself a massage, then tap your skin with a towel before getting dressed so the oil doesn't get on your clothing.

6. **A Glass of Warm Water.** A glass of warm water in the morning can help with your morning elimination. It's very healthy to go to the bathroom first thing in the morning, each day.

7. **Joint Warm-Ups and a Few Gentle Yoga Postures.** This will prepare the body for the movements you'll be doing throughout your day. This easeful physical activity can also help with your morning elimination and help ground you in the present moment.

8. **A Walk Outside.** Even if you walk for just a short distance, going outside connects you to the freshness of the morning's air. It can help you wake up and feel the qualities of the elements supporting you.

9. **Pranayama.** You can choose a pranayama that suits your own constitution and how you are feeling today. If you exhibiting signs of imbalanced vata, choose a pranayama for calming and grounding. If you are kaphic, start with some deep breaths and then choose a warming breath. If you are predominantly showing signs of pitta imbalance, choose a pitty pacifying breath.

The morning routine allows you to start your day from a clean, fresh, and healthy place. It supports your immune system and prepares your mind and body for the activity and work that you'll be doing the rest of the day. It's so supportive to your health to give yourself this attention in the morning, after you've been asleep so that you make a smooth and mindful transition into your day.

ESSENTIAL

Mouth care is important especially because it's needed for your intake of food and digestion. A very healthy tip for the morning and evening routine is to swish sesame oil all around in the mouth for a few moments, and then spit it out. This supports the health of your entire mouth, especially the gums.

Once you are used to cleansing the sense organs, the tongue, nose, eyes, ears, and skin, that part of the morning routine will only take about twenty minutes. By doing the morning routine, you are starting your day by creating the conditions for you to be in balance. Throughout the day you'll make choices in the dance of life to stay in balance, and starting off the morning this way will make it easier for you to move through your life with ease and clarity.

Following Nature's Clock

The natural clock has the qualities of the doshas, just as you do. The hours between 2 A.M. and 6 A.M. are vata time; 6 A.M. to 10 A.M. is kapha time; 10 A.M. to 2 P.M. is pitta time; 2 to 6 P.M. is vata time; 6 to 10 P.M. is kapha time; 10 P.M. to 2 A.M. is pitta time. During these times you are affected by those qualities. When your constitution is the same as the time of day, then those qualities will be heightened for you. Everyone is affected by nature's clock, however, so there are general guidelines of when to wake up, have your heaviest meal, and go to bed.

Keeping a Schedule

Waking up naturally is best. Allowing natural light to come into your bedroom so you wake up to it keeps you in sync with nature. Ayurveda recommends you get up before 6 A.M. (or sunrise) so that you aren't waking up during kapha time.

Kapha time, 6 A.M.–10 A.M., is a great time to be doing your morning routine because the earth and water qualities of kapha support lubrication of the joints and movement. If you are predominantly kapha, it will be supportive to you to include some kind of activity in the morning (between 6 A.M. and 8 A.M.), such as asanas or a brisk walk or run before you have breakfast. Eat a light breakfast around 8 A.M., and then begin work around 9 A.M. For pitta, start with a calming morning routine, and before breakfast do asanas or run. Eat breakfast around 7 or 8 A.M., and then begin your regular work activities around 9 A.M. after eating a leisurely breakfast. If you are predominantly vata, keep the entire morning calm as you do your routine, and eat your breakfast slowly. Begin your workday around 10 A.M.

After kapha time is pitta time. It's best to eat your heaviest meal at lunchtime, when nature has pitta qualities. For all doshas this is the time to eat the heaviest meal. If you are predominantly pitta, be mindful of your interactions with others and the activities you do between 10 A.M. and 2 P.M. This is when your fiery qualities can be most aggravated by the time of day.

Vata time is 2 P.M.–6 P.M. For pitta and kapha types, this is a great time to be engaged in work and mental activities. If you are primarily vata, be mindful during these hours. Do what you need to feel grounded. You may need to take breaks from work at this time. Take time to meditate. If you can, take a nap. Drink some hot tea. Take time to relax during these hours.

Kapha time is 6 P.M.–10 P.M. This is the perfect time to have a leisurely dinner. Begin to unwind from the day. Allow the kapha energy to ground you and prepare you for bedtime. For all types, it's best to go to sleep by or around 10 P.M., while still in kapha time.

A Naturally Healthy Way of Eating

The foods you eat and your relationship to food are important factors in how healthy you are. Often in modern Western culture, food isn't seen as the medicine or the nourishment that it truly is. Your body needs the nutrients found in whole foods, and it can't thrive on a diet that consists primarily of processed food. Also, your attitude toward the food as you prepare and eat it makes a difference.

How to Know What to Eat

You can use the qualities of your constitution and the qualities of foods as a guide for choosing what to eat and at what time of year. You want to regain and maintain balance in relation to your own constitution and the season. Ayurveda lists certain foods, spices, and tastes that support each dosha and combinations of doshas.

You can use various Ayurvedic resources to compare and learn about which foods are good for which types. See Appendix B for a list of resources. And once you get used to Ayurveda, you will also be able to use your own common sense in the kitchen. You will remember that like increases like and opposites balance. You will know your constitution, and you will be

able to assess which foods will be most supportive to yo[...]
seasons.

QUOTE

> At the end of the day everything boils down to qualitie[...]
> is moist and fatty and is a wonderful food for vata cons[...]
> tends to be dry. Cucumbers are a cooling veggie and s[...]
> body type, which tends to run hot, while dry figs, which [...]
> support the moist nature of the kapha constitution. —Danny Arguetty,
> Nutrition and Health Counselor

The tastes are an additional concept around eating that is unique to Ayurveda. Depending on your constitution, there are recommendations for which tastes to favor and avoid.

▼ 5.2: DOSHAS AND THE TASTES

Dosha	Tastes to Favor	Tastes to Avoid
Vata	sweet, sour, salty	bitter, pungent, astringent
Pitta	sweet, bitter, astringent	sour, salty, pungent
Kapha	pungent, bitter, astringent	sweet, sour, salty

The doshas—vata, pitta, kapha—have the qualities of their associated elements, and the elements produce or have tastes inherent in them. Vata—space and air—contains bitter, pungent, and astringent tastes. That is why those are the tastes to avoid for vata, and vata should favor sweet, sour, and salty tastes, which are the tastes inherent in kapha (the water and earth elements) that vata doesn't inherently possess. In the same way, pitta is of fire and water, whose associated tastes are sour, salty, and pungent. For this reason, since Ayurveda instructs that opposites balance, pitta types will favor the tastes that aren't naturally strong in their constitution: sweet, bitter, and astringent. And kapha is of water and earth elements, which have the sweet, sour, and salty tastes. So kapha types will do well to favor pungent, bitter, and astringent tastes. It's the same principle throughout Ayurveda: balance the qualities to create the conditions for health.

w Much to Eat

So that your body can process the food that you ingest, it's important to be mindful of how much you eat at your meals. A general rule is to imagine you are filling your stomach one-third full of food, one-third full of warm water, and leaving one-third empty.

QUESTION

How do I know how big my stomach is?
Your stomach can shrink and also expand. It is typically suggested that the appropriate amount of food for you as an individual will be the amount you can hold in your two cupped hands.

This might feel like an unusually small amount of food, based on what you are used to eating. If that's the case, then over time reduce your food intake at meals. It's likely that your stomach has stretched to accommodate the excess food you've been eating, so it will need some time to resume its natural size. Because of this, if you reduce your amount of food at meals, you may think you are still hungry. Try to resist the urge to keep overeating. It can help to drink warm water with lemon throughout the day to stay hydrated and also to curb your appetite.

You will likely notice that when you begin to eat whole, unprocessed foods for your type, you will be satisfied with less food than what you might be used to. Your body will respond and be satisfied because it will be receiving what it needs for nutrition.

In the end it is most important to eat as consciously as possible and trust in how you feel. Your body will let you know what it needs and how much it needs if you cultivate the practices of conscious eating.

Enjoyment of Food

Make cooking and eating a process that is worth celebrating. Acknowledge that other people's work has gone into the harvesting and preparing of the food in front of you. Remember that what you're about to enjoy grew beautifully from the earth and other people have worked so that the food can arrive at your grocery store or market. Before you cook and eat, take time to be grateful. Cultivating this attitude sends a positive energy into the food and acknowledges what it took to get it to you. It also helps you relax and prepare to eat, which can help prevent overeating.

WAYS TO NOTICE AND APPRECIATE YOUR FOOD

- Look at the food: notice the colors and shapes.
- Inhale and take a moment to appreciate the scents.
- After taking a bite, slowly chew and pay attention to the tastes.
- As you swallow, imagine the food traveling into your body, carrying the nutrients and energy you use throughout your day.
- Take a breath between each bite. Savor the meal.

As you cook or prepare meals, fill your food with healing and loving intention. Thoughts, emotions, and words carry vibrations. The food will pick up and carry the vibrations you put into it. Fill your food with nourishing, healing vibration. Enjoy the process of cooking; enjoy the process of eating.

Cultivate Self-Awareness and Compassion

Becoming aware of what you say, think, feel, and do is an essential part of healthy living. This is true for many reasons. At the very basic level, you must be able to observe yourself in order to know what's working, what's not working, and how to create balance. Practice noticing what you do, how you do it, and how that affects the way you experience health and your life. By observing yourself—your thoughts, your reactions, your energy levels, how you treat others, how you treat yourself, what you eat, what you do for exercise, how you feel about exercise, etc.—you can learn what's supporting your health and what's detracting from your being able to live a life that is naturally healthful and beautiful. Once you can notice how you are, Ayurveda can give you the tools and guidance you need.

When you observe yourself, practice observing with compassion. When you notice something about you that you think you want to change, notice it with compassion. For example, if you notice you don't eat well all day and then you are so hungry you eat a whole bag of candy, just notice that.

Then, notice if your tendency is to want to mentally punish yourself, thinking you've done something "bad." See if you can turn that around. Instead of thinking you've done something wrong, ask yourself if you eat bags of candy often enough whether it's a behavior you'd like to change. If so, that's a good thing to notice: this is something you would like to change. You have the power to do that, and you don't have to mentally punish yourself. Instead, educate yourself about what would be a healthier, satisfying, sweet snack.

ESSENTIAL

Thinking negative thoughts is just as unhealthy for you as eating unhealthy food. Negative emotions, thoughts, and feelings move from energetic dis-ease to mental and physical disease. It's just as important to learn new ways of working with your mental and energetic bodies as it is to learn new ways of taking care of your physical body.

If you notice you often turn to candy or other sweets that aren't very healthy for you, there are new habits you can create. Because Ayurveda helps you create a life of balance, you will notice that one effect of living in balance is that you'll have less cravings (if any). A reason to start creating balance is that you'll crave healthy foods and know which foods will satisfy and nourish you. Bags of candy are actually much less satisfying than healthy meals and healthy treats, which you'll soon discover! It's important as a first step to notice the habits you want to change, have compassion for yourself, and then look to another way of doing things—such as Ayurveda.

How to Cultivate Compassion

You cannot feel compassion for others if you do not feel it for yourself. Any parts of yourself you reject, you will reject in others. Parts of yourself that you repress will trigger you when you see it in others. The more compassionate awareness you can have for all aspects of who you are, the more you can have that for others. Honest compassion for yourself and others is a recipe for personal and global healing.

To cultivate compassion for yourself, be gentle with yourself. Spend time in meditation allowing thoughts to arise so you can see what they are. When you meditate, you sit in stillness. As thoughts arise, notice that they are there. Compassionately notice whatever they are. And, then, allow them to drift by. Focus on your breath, the present moment of the breath flowing in and out, without your needing to control it. As thoughts arise, again, notice them. Do not judge them. And then allow them to float by like the clouds in the sky. Compassionately acknowledge your thoughts, without judgment and without attaching to them during your meditation. This is a way to cultivate compassion for yourself.

QUOTE

The highest form of spiritual practice is self-observation without judgment. —Swami Kripalu

Acknowledge Suffering

To cultivate compassion for yourself and others, call to mind the idea that everyone knows what it is like to suffer. You have experienced suffering in your life—you've been hurt, disappointed, and/or grieved the loss of a loved one. Everyone has. This suffering is a universal experience. If you recognize that you have suffered and how you deal with it affects how you act in the world, you can recognize that others are suffering, too, and are doing the best they can.

Being compassionate doesn't mean you have to be friends with everyone you meet. It does mean that you'll do your best, even with someone you can't bear to spend time with, to honor the light that is in them. It doesn't mean you compromise your well-being by trying to fix or heal them. If you can't be friends with them, it's okay. You can acknowledge that to yourself, create a boundary by not spending time with the person, and still know he is suffering, or has suffered, and is doing his best in the world just as you are.

Metta Meditation

Another way to cultivate compassion is metta meditation. To do this, get in a comfortable, seated position as you would for seated meditation. Close your eyes and get grounded. Feel your sitting bones rooted into the cushion that you're seated on. Take a deep inhale and a long exhale. Do this deep breathing a few more times. Then, be still. Watch your breath for a few exhales. Then, follow these steps, with an open heart:

1. Say this silently to yourself: "May I be happy. May I be healthy. May I be safe."
2. Call to mind someone whom you love dearly. Hold this person in your heart, and silently send this wish to her: "May you be happy. May you be healthy. May you be safe."
3. Call to mind someone you don't know very well, whose path you cross now and then. Send this heartfelt wish silently to that person: "May you be happy. May you be healthy. May you be safe."
4. Call to mind everyone in your neighborhood, village, or city, and silently send this wish to them: "May you be happy. May you be healthy. May you be safe."
5. Call to mind someone with whom you have a conflict. Knowing he is suffering, silently send him this wish: "May you be happy. May you be healthy. May you be safe."
6. Call to mind all the service-minded people in the world who in any way, large or small, serve others in their work or in their lives. Send them this wish: "May you be happy. May you be healthy. May you be safe."
7. Hold in your heart all beings everywhere, and send out this wish: "May you be happy. May you be healthy. May you be safe."
8. Take a moment in silence. Breathe. Notice how you feel. Acknowledge the meditative space you've been in and take a moment to transition back into your day.

Metta meditation helps you cultivate compassion for yourself first and then give it out to the rest of the world. This practice helps you really feel and see that everyone and everything is connected and wants to be happy, healthy, and secure.

Ease Into Bedtime

Getting a good night's sleep is so important for your mental, physical, and energetic bodies. Your entire being benefits from sleep. Modern medical studies show you need seven to nine hours of sleep to regulate your metabolism. Ayurveda has known for millennia how vital sleep is. During sleep you digest what you've eaten and what your senses have taken in during your waking hours. It's an essential part of your daily cycle. As with all parts of your daily cycle it will help you and your nervous system if you transition mindfully from one phase to the next. So rather than work until late at night and then konk out at bedtime from exhaustion and overwork, you could stop work earlier and have an easeful, nice transition from your working hours into your sleeping hours. Creating this sense of calm and ease, making space between work and sleep, gives your body the signal that there's plenty of time for rest and sleep.

Why Do You Stay Up Late?

Decide ahead of time what time you would like to go to sleep. Ayurveda recommends going to bed by or around 10 P.M. That might not be possible for you. Perhaps 11 P.M. is a more reasonable goal. Being intentional about your schedule helps create structure for important self-care routines.

ESSENTIAL

If you want to have better health, you have to do something different. If you stay up too late, examine why and what you're doing. Are you taking time to wind down, or are you working, worrying, or partying? Watch what you do at those hours, and ask yourself if that's something you're willing to change.

Maybe you think you wouldn't be tired enough to go to bed at 10 P.M. See if that's true. See what happens if you give yourself time to unwind. It's true there is so much one could do each day. Ask yourself if it is worth compromising your health for these other things.

Time to Unwind

Instead of watching TV or working late, what could you be doing for yourself and your health between the hours of 8 P.M. and 10 P.M.? If you were to go to bed around 10 P.M., you would start unwinding around 7 P.M. or 8 P.M. That means, when it's 7 P.M. or 8 P.M., you stop engaging in work and stimulating activities. Have some soothing tea. Read a meditative or inspirational book. Give yourself an oil massage. Take a hot bath. Write a fun letter. Spend time with your family or your friends, not watching television or on the computer. Face paint each other. Go for a night walk. Read poetry. Knit. For a couple of hours, give yourself nourishing, relaxing time. Then slip into bed by 10 P.M., without having the speedy work or Internet communication still buzzing around in your mind. The benefit is that you get some nourishing time into your day and you transition with nature into the kapha time of night from 10 P.M. to 2 A.M.

CHAPTER 6

Rediscover Your Relationship to Food

Can you imagine how you'd feel if you allowed yourself to sit down for every meal, focused on the pleasure of eating and enjoying the moment? Imagine what it would feel like if you were to chew slowly and savor the tastes of every bite. What if you were to learn that making time to sit down and enjoy eating, whether alone or in good company, is not a frivolous way of passing time? In fact how you eat, coupled with what you eat, is a key factor in a healthy lifestyle.

Food Worth Believing In

You've heard of the placebo effect? It is when doctors give patients sugar pills and tell them that those pills are medication. There has been substantial evidence that shows placebos can work. In other words, although there's nothing chemically healing in the pill, the power of the patient's belief creates or advances his own healing process. Such placebo studies are one form of validation and confirmation of the power of belief on health and healing. This is an example of modern science's use of the phenomenon that Ayurveda has held and experienced as truth for millennia: that your belief has real and powerful healing potential.

If you can believe in the efficacy of a pill that your doctor prescribes for you, could you also strongly believe that whole foods, natural herbs, spices, oils, and yoga postures that are recommended for you will help you sustain optimal health?

QUOTE

Eat food. Not too much. Mostly plants. That, more or less, is the short answer to the supposedly incredibly complicated and confusing question of what we humans should eat in order to be maximumly healthy. —Michael Pollan

The first steps toward remembering your natural connection to food and its vital role in your health are:

- Become intentional about what foods you eat. Choose whole, natural foods, organic and locally grown when possible.
- Bring the joy back into eating and cooking. Take pleasure in noticing that whole foods are rich in color, diverse in texture, and varied in their delicious tastes.
- Believe in the healing and nourishing power of natural, whole foods. They really are what your body, mind, and spirit need to thrive.

Perhaps one of the biggest challenges for you will be not to make processed and adulterated foods a routine part of your diet. If you can shift from eating processed foods to natural and whole foods, you won't have to worry about looking at labels and trying to decipher which meals are good for you and how much surreptitiously added sugar is in each bite. If you have to spend time trying to understand the label, it's a good sign you don't need to be eating that item.

Michael Pollan's *In Defense of Food* is written in a very simple, engaging voice, and he explains very clearly the health benefits of a whole foods diet. He also explains why our culture has become fixated on calories and ingredients rather than on the benefits of just enjoying and eating real food. The truth is, if you spend your time in the produce section, the bulk foods section (for foods such as lentils, nuts, and seeds), and reveling in the seasonal varieties of all-natural whole foods, there isn't any "nutritional value" you have to be worrying about or trying to understand. You can believe in whole foods; they are crafted from nature and have in them what you need.

Ayurveda explains how to best choose foods for you based on the qualities you find in nature and in yourself.

Savor the Moment

If you enjoy and appreciate what you're eating while you're eating it, you enhance your body's ability to digest and absorb what your body needs. Create a safe, loving, happy, and relaxed atmosphere at mealtimes. With a very busy lifestyle, it may be difficult to be in a relaxed mind-set when you eat. You may feel you must keep working while you eat, or you may keep walking around the kitchen when you eat. If this is true for you, start by just slowing it down a little bit, sitting down, and taking some deep breaths before you take a bite. This really might not be easy for you. You might think, "Oh, well, that can't be so important, it's just important to know what to eat." Not so. How you eat is important for digestion, elimination, and absorption.

See if you can make this change: slow down and sit down to focus on eating. It might take some real willpower, and it might mean you mark it in your day planner. See if you can do this for a few days, consistently, at least for two meals a day, and notice what difference occurs for you around eating and in your life. To do this, ahead of time, decide which two meals you will spend a half hour sitting down for and relaxing. Really decide, ahead of time, that this is important. Make that commitment to yourself. This might be a big change for you if you're used to eating energy bars on the run. You will notice the benefits, more and more over time. And Ayurveda gives you encouragement to really take pleasure in your thoughts around food and eating, for your health and longevity.

ESSENTIAL

The importance of sitting down to eat cannot be overemphasized because in our culture it's no longer thought of as a priority. Remember, this is your time to give fuel to your body. What could be more important to prioritize? You have the opportunity to really make a difference for yourself by adding "time to eat" into your routine.

It doesn't have to be a chore to learn how to make good choices: it can be fun and nurturing. Think of it as a way for you to experience more joy in life, every single time you eat, by savoring the effects that food has on your senses of sight, smell, touch, and taste. You really deserve to enjoy your meals, and when you slow down and eat in a way that works for your constitution, you will be able to use food as one of the ways to balance your mood and your energy.

The All-Purpose Secret Ingredient: Good Vibrations

Your all-purpose secret ingredient will cost you nothing, and you never have to go the store to get more of it: it's your energetic vibration. The way you are feeling mentally and emotionally, coupled with your intentions during cooking, is transferred into the food as you prepare it. To use this to your great advantage, as you prepare meals, imagine transferring loving, healing, supportive energy into the food. Often people already do this, especially when cooking for someone they love: they automatically transfer their loving energy into the food. Other times, people are so busy and rushed that the hurried energy or frustrated energy gets transferred into the food. You are always transmitting vibrations of energy, so be sure to transmit good vibrations into whatever you are going to eat and serve to others.

Eat in Moderation

This isn't news, right? Eating in moderation just makes sense. Ayurveda recommends that you eat slowly, chew your food well, and enjoy the tastes. If you slow down and savor what you're eating, it will help you eat less food: you will feel the satisfaction of the smells and tastes, and you won't be shoveling it in mindlessly mouthful after mouthful. Oftentimes if you don't pay attention while you're eating, you could even forget if you have eaten, or soon after you've eaten you may still think you're hungry because you weren't paying attention when you ate. It will help you eat in moderation if you take your time and allow yourself to enjoy the food. Choosing the right foods for your constitution will also help you feel satisfied with appropriate amounts: the tastes and qualities will balance your hunger.

How Much to Eat

A good rule of thumb is to eat about two handfuls of food per meal. To imagine how full your stomach should be after a meal, imagine it as one-third filled with food, one-third filled with warm water, and one-third empty. During your meal, sip warm (or room temperature) water.

Overeating

If you overeat, your stomach will expand, and then it will feel empty even with the appropriate amount of food inside. That will cause you to eat more, and then your stomach will expand more, and so goes the pattern. Eating the right amount is important because you want to give yourself enough of the fuel you need, while being careful not to overload your system with more food than it can digest at a time.

If you notice you don't feel full with two handfuls of food as your guideline, try sipping lemon water throughout the day. Or, if there's a time of day you tend to want to snack, prepare a cup of tea around that time before the hunger strikes. Tulsi tea is a great pick-me-up and can be a mood enhancer and stress reliever. There are many varieties of tulsi tea available, and some are mixed with other teas for a different kind of flavor and effect. If you want a decaffeinated tea, make sure your tulsi tea is not blended with a caffeinated tea.

If you have high vata energy, you may notice your appetite is variable. When you aren't hungry for breakfast or dinner, drink a cup of warm milk with a teaspoon of cardamom. This soothing and grounding drink will help balance the cool and dry qualities of vata and give you some nourishment so you won't feel starved later.

Tastes Help You Determine What to Eat

An important and unique aspect of Ayurveda is the role that tastes play in determining what foods to eat. Ayurveda describes six possible tastes that you can experience (sweet, sour, salty, pungent, bitter, and astringent). Each taste is described in terms of the same elements and qualities of the doshas and the natural elements (such as heating, cooling, dry). Each taste, because of its qualities, will help balance different doshas and affect the digestive fire differently. As always, remember that like increases like and opposites balance. So you'll want to choose tastes with qualities that balance (are opposite to) the elemental qualities of your constitution and elements outside. Of course, be in consultation with your Ayurvedic specialist because she will also take into consideration what she learns about your digestion and what else is going on in your body, mind, and life. That way she can recommend supportive ways to use the tastes in your diet.

What if I don't have a good sense of taste?
To enhance your sense of taste, practice bringing your focus to what you are eating. Don't create distractions with television or phone calls. After taking a bite, close your eyes to help you focus on the process of eating. Always chew your food very well to get the digestive enzymes flowing and to give you more time to experience tastes.

The following information about the tastes provides general guidelines to help you understand the value of tastes and their qualities. Remember, you are unique, and your needs shift with time, seasons, and changes in your life. Talk with your Ayurvedic specialist for more guidance in understanding how the elements are showing up in you and which tastes would be great for you to favor and which to avoid.

The following is a table that shows the six tastes and their associated elements.

Taste	Elements
Sweet	earth and water
Sour	earth and fire
Salty	fire and water
Pungent	air and fire
Bitter	air and ether
Astringent	air and earth

Each taste has more than one effect on the body and mind. **Rasa** is the actual taste. **Virya** is the potency in regard to its energy of warming or cooling to the system. Tastes that are more predominant in sweet, bitter, and astringent have a cooling effect. Tastes that are predominant in pungent, salty, and sour have a heating effect.

Vipaka is the postdigestive effect, which may show a different quality than either the rasa or virya and is often very important. The postdigestive effect will become how the foods affect your tissues. There are three types: sweet, sour, pungent. These effects are consistent with how each taste affects you.

- Sweet vipaka comes from sweet and salty taste.
- Sour vipaka comes from sour tastes.
- Pungent vipaka comes from pungent, astringent, and bitter tastes.

Once you become accustomed to the concept of tastes in this way, you will begin to think of food in a whole new light. Soon, you will naturally think of the tastes according to their qualities, just as you begin to see yourself and the world around you in terms of qualities. In this way, you'll see how everything in life is connected.

Tastes for Vata

Remember, the qualities associated with vata are cold, dry, light, and mobile. So, you want to ground vata's energy and balance it with these qualities: warm, moist, and heavy. The tastes that are best for vata are sweet, salty, and sour.

Sweet to Ground Vata

Sweet taste is made up of the elements earth and water, and the sweet taste has moist and heavy qualities both short-term and long-term. These qualities are wonderful for balancing vata's light, mobile, and dry qualities. Sweet has a slightly cooling effect on the digestive system, but just enough to give you a sense of feeling full or satisfied.

Sour's Warming and Heavy Support

Sour's elements are earth and fire, which means sour is grounding and heating, with some moisture. The heating quality of sour helps kindle the digestive fire, making this taste very supportive for vata. The warming and grounding effects stay with the body beyond the process of digestion, which is also very balancing for vata.

These qualities affect the mind, not just the body. So, for example, the grounding quality of sour will create feelings of steadiness and support counteracting vata's tendency toward anxiety and fear.

Salty Benefits for Vata

The salty taste comprises fire and water. Its initial effects on the system are heating and moistening, which help to balance vata's cool and dry qualities. The fiery element of the salty taste supports digestion, which is very supportive for vata types whose appetite can be variable and whose coolness and dryness affect the digestive fire.

Long-term, the salty taste has a sweet vipaka, which means its postdigestive effects are of those elements of the sweet taste—earth and water. Therefore, long-term, the effects are moistening and grounding (excellent for vata).

Which Tastes Are Less Favorable for Vata?

Certain tastes are less favorable than others for vata. You don't have to avoid these tastes altogether; just be mindful about how often you choose these tastes if you're working with vata imbalance. For instance, if you're feeling well and if you're out to eat and want to try something on the menu that has the taste that's not the most supportive to your constitution, it's okay. You can incorporate some of the less favorable tastes into your meal. It may throw you a little off-kilter, but being in balance is a process; you will fluctuate. While it's best to do as many things as possible to support your health most of the time, there's no need to be incredibly rigid and fearful around the guidelines. When deciding what to eat, take into consideration not just the tastes but also the food temperature, the weather outside, the time of day, and what else is going on in your life to help you decide how much support you're needing in the moment to balance vata.

A Little Pungent Is Okay for Vata

The elements that make up the taste pungent are air and fire, and pungent's vipaka is also pungent. So, the light and airy qualities will be its short- and longer-term effect. Vata doesn't need more air or lightness to stay in the body so that's why this taste is not highly recommended for vata.

ESSENTIAL

If, lately, your skin is very dry, you are feeling anxious and cold, and it's also fall or wintertime—vata time of year—focus on tastes that don't have airy or dry qualities. Remember that choosing what you put into your body is one of the most direct ways you can positively (or adversely) affect how you're feeling.

Because fire is also an element of pungent, some pungency is all right for vata. Vata could use the heat. To make pungency work for vata, be sure to eat other foods or tastes that are grounding and moistening (to balance the air element).

Bitter Is of the Same Elements as Vata

Bitter is made of the elements of ether and air, and for this reason it's not recommended for vata types. Its vipaka is cooling. So, some bitter taste will be fine, as all tastes are necessary. You just need to balance it. For example, kale has a bitter taste. So, to make this green food supportive to vata, cook the kale so that it's very warm and moist, oil it well using ghee, and toss in some salt and pumpkin seeds.

Astringent Is Too Drying for Vata

Astringent's elements are earth and air, and its light and drying effects are both short- and long-term because air is an element that is part of its virya and vipaka. Its vipaka is cooling. Over time it's very drying. Astringent tastes are not thought of as supportive to digestion, and vata needs digestive support. With all the wonderful whole and natural foods available to support vata, it's best to limit your use of astringent tastes when cooking for those with a predominance of vata.

Tastes for Pitta

Remember that pitta's elements are fire and water. Keep in mind that the qualities of the elements that make up pitta include hot, oily, light, mobile, and liquid. When choosing tastes to incorporate into your meal, you'll want to balance these qualities with their opposites.

Sweet for Pitta

Sweet's elements are earth and water. Its virya is cooling, which is a great balance for pitta. Pitta types tend to have a strong appetite and digestion, so the cooling aspect of sweet can help soothe and calm the hunger a little bit. The cooling quality also can help pitta stay balanced and not slide into judgmentalism, anger, and jealousy.

As a rule, sweet's vipaka is also sweet, which means it has long-term grounding, moistening, and slightly cooling effects—very good for balancing pitta's mobile, light, and hot qualities.

ESSENTIAL

Bitter Cools Down Pitta

Bitter is a great taste for cooling pitta. Bitter's elements are air and ether, which makes it the coolest of the tastes. Its virya is cooling, and even though its vipaka is pungent, it is recommended to help balance pitta.

Also, in small amounts, for everyone, the bitter taste clears and opens the mind, helping you to see things just as they are. When you begin to see situations in your life for all they offer, the easeful part and the difficult parts, you can make choices from a better place than you can if you're not seeing so clearly.

Astringent Pacifies Pitta

Astrigent's elements are air and earth. These combine to have a cooling virya, which is wonderful for pitta. Its vipaka is pungent, which means that the airy quality continues and the light and dry qualities have a nice effect for pitta.

Tastes That Aggravate Pitta

Because pitta is of earth and fire, when cooking for predominantly pitta types (and on hot days) choose tastes that aren't heating. The following tastes are not the best to use when cooking for pitta.

Sour Creates Heat

Sour's elements are earth and fire. Its virya and vipaka are heating, which means that it heats up during digestion and continues to have heating qualities after digestion. This isn't what pitta needs. Too much heat for pitta will aggravate the body as well as the mind, potentially leading you to feel jealous, judgmental, angry, and irritated. If you do have sour in your meal, balance it with other tastes that can help counteract the heating effects.

Salt Is Heating, Then Mild

Salt's elements are fire and water. With its heating virya, it can be aggravating to pitta. Salt's vipaka is sweet, which means it cools down after digestion. Sweet is a grounding taste that is good for pitta's diet, so some salty taste in moderation would be fine for pitta. Every person is different, though, so take note of how it affects you. You will notice for yourself how often the taste of salt is okay for you.

Prepare Pungent for Pitta?

Not a good idea. Of all the tastes, pungent is the hottest, with elements of air and fire. You don't want to make a pungent dish in the middle of summertime for lunch if you're already experiencing a predominance of pitta in your constitution. If you serve pungent dishes to someone who is predominantly pitta, you really want to balance it with other tastes or balancing foods. The taste pungent has a vipaka that is pungent: the qualities it engenders even after digestion are heating, light, and dry.

Tastes for Kapha

Kapha's elements are water and earth. Kapha is stable, damp, and cold. When choosing tastes for kapha, the best tastes are those that will have heating and slightly drying qualities. These balance the heavy and moist kapha qualities.

Pungent to Heat Kapha

Pungent, as the hottest of the tastes, is a great match for a kapha type. It will help with digestion and an overall heating of the body. Pungent's elements are air and fire, which makes it hot, dry, and mobile.

Pungent's vipaka is still pungent, so the heating and drying effects are powerful and long-lasting. That's good news for kapha!

Since childhood is the kapha time of life, pungent is a taste to think about adding when you are preparing children's meals. Adding the pungent taste can be done as easily as flavoring dishes with garlic and onions.

You Can Lighten Up with Bitter

Bitter taste has light and dry qualities, so it's a good taste for kapha types. Its elements are air and ether, which means it also has the quality of coolness. Even though kapha is already cool, bitter taste is very supportive because it's drying and light from beginning to end—balancing the water and earth elements of kapha. Its vipaka is pungent, so the long-term qualities are very supportive to kapha: light, dry, heating.

Astringent Works for Kapha

Astringent and kapha are both made up of earth as one of their two elements. Astringent is a good balance for kapha because astringent's other element is air. Kapha's is water. The air element creates lightness and dryness, a great balance for kapha's water element.

Like bitter, astringent has a pungent vipaka. So, at first, astringent will have a cooling effect on the body and on digestion, and then its postdigestive qualities are heating, dry, and light. That's the opposite and thus a good support to kapha.

Tastes That Don't Support Kapha

Kapha is made of the stable element earth and the lubricating element water. If you are feeling the effects of the kapha dosha, you don't want to choose tastes that are going to increase the heavy and liquid qualities. This can cause depression, lethargy, weight gain, and possessiveness. So, be mindful of the following tastes in your diet. If you choose them, then be sure to also have some lighter, drying, and heating tastes/foods, as well.

Kapha Doesn't Need Sweetness

A kapha individual can be a very grounded and nurturing personality. He doesn't need more sweetness; he already has a wonderful amount. Sweet's elements are the same as kapha's: earth and water as its virya and vipaka. These two elements together help a body bulk up with weight gain when eaten in excess and can lead to inertia. A little bit of sweet is fine at the end of a meal to help you feel satisfied, but for kapha types it's best to not plan your meals to include a lot of this taste.

Sour and Kapha

Sour has a warming effect on the body, which could be a nice balance to kapha. However, sour in general has a heavy, grounded, and moist feel to it. Its elements are earth and fire. And the groundedness and unctuous qualities of sour could be too much for kapha. If you do want to include sour in your meal—for you, your kapha friend, or a child—it would be best to find a way to balance it using other tastes or foods.

Salty Taste Shares Kapha's Heaviness

One of the effects of the salty taste is that it helps the body retain water. Kapha, being of earth and water, does not need help retaining water. Extra salt in the kapha diet will create more of what kapha already has. Though the elements of salt's intial taste are fire and water, which means the fire will initially feel heating for kapha, salt's vipaka is sweet: very heavy and moist. That means, postdigestion, salt's qualities are earth and water—increasing what kapha already has naturally, taking it to excess.

Examples of Foods and Their Tastes

Ayurveda has observed and documented the qualities of the tastes, and the categorizations are to help choose what's best for you. Because such a treatment of taste is not usually considered in the Western view of a healthy diet, you may not be used to recognizing the tastes in the foods you eat.

Taste	Foods
Sweet	sugar, rice, milk
Sour	lemon, vinegar, pickles
Salty	salt, seaweed, salted snacks (nuts, popcorn)
Pungent	onions, garlic, hot pepper, ginger
Bitter	green, leafy vegetables; neem; aloe vera; black or green tea
Astringent	chickpeas, lentils, peels of fruit, turmeric, cranberries

Each taste, because of its qualities, has a different effect on your body and mind. The easiest way to remember the effects is to think in terms of qualities. If you are running hot, choose tastes that are cooling. If you're feeling sluggish and lethargic, choose tastes that are associated with fire to add some kick and to stimulate energy in your system.

Spice Mixes to Customize Your Meal

Masala is a term used to describe a spice blend or spice mixture. You can use spice mixtures to enhance the flavor of food, to improve digestion, and for their therapeutic properties (such as carminative, alterative, diuretic, or analgesic). Using the right spices in your diet will help you maintain strong digestive fire, reduce toxins, and bring balance to the doshas.

How to Cook with Masalas

One of the best ways to cook with masalas is to sauté the blends in some ghee (clarified butter) or oil. The ghee or oil helps to extract the flavors and aromas of these spices while releasing the natural oils, which contain many of the therapeutic components. Once you mix the spices in ghee or oil, add vegetables or your choice of other food to the mixture and sauté. Masalas can also be added to soups, stews, rice, or kitchari.

You can customize spice blends so they will help pacify any doshic imbalance or vikruti and so that they suit your taste. For example, a person who is experiencing high kapha may want to use a kapha-reducing masala to prepare his or her food. Here are masala recipes for each dosha.

Masala for Vata Type

2 tablespoons cumin
1 tablespoon turmeric
1 tablespoon fennel
1 teaspoon asafoetida

1 teaspoon ginger
1 teaspoon sesame seeds
½ teaspoon mineral salt

Masala for Pitta Type

2 tablespoons coriander
1 tablespoon cumin
1 tablespoon turmeric
1 tablespoon fennel

1 teaspoon cardamom
1 teaspoon raw sugar
¼ teaspoon clove

Masala for Kapha Type

1 tablespoon turmeric
1 tablespoon coriander
1 tablespoon fennel

1 teaspoon cinnamon
1 teaspoon cumin
1 teaspoon ginger

To save time, make several servings of these masalas ahead of time, and keep them for up to six months. Have them nearby with your other spices so you can easily reach for them when you're cooking. Here are more tips when making spice masalas:

- It's best to use the powdered form of the spices. If you can, buy whole spices in bulk and grind them using a spice grinder or a mortar and pestle.
- Organic and nonirradiated spices are of the best quality.
- Store masalas in a sealed container in a cool, dark place.

Spice blends are delicious, nutritious, and fun to use. Because they have an array of therapeutic benefits for the body, mind, and senses, it's no wonder that spices in times of trade have been valued as highly as gold.

CHAPTER 7

Understanding Vata

Vata is made up of air and space. When vata is out of balance, a variety of uncomfortable symptoms can occur, from dry mouth to constipation. And the longer vata is left unchecked, the more wear and tear your body will experience from the inside out. When you keep vata in balance, there are so many wonderful mental and physical processes it supports, from expansive and creative thinking to proper biological functions.

What Is Vata?

Vata is made up of the elements of air and space. This combination of elements is the force behind many vital functions in the body, including the functioning of the heart and circulatory system. Vata also helps fan the fire of digestion and aids in elimination. Its energy is necessary for the workings of the mind and intellect. Through its vital role in the functions of the heart, mind, gut, and intellect, vata helps you experience your deepest wisdom and brightest knowing.

Vata is located in and as the space in the open cavities of the body, such as the spaces in between bones and joints—particularly in the lower back, pelvic area, and hips. Its primary site is the colon.

Vital Life-Force Energy: Prana

Prana is vital life-force energy. It's likened to the concept of *chi* in Chinese medicine and *qi* in Japanese culture. The Western medical system doesn't address prana. This is a main cause for so many people seeking complementary treatments: most people are noticing that they aren't healing well because something is not being seen. What's not being seen is the whole person. For complete healing, the whole person must be examined: the mental, emotional, and energetic components of the self. Otherwise, complete physical well-being is not sustainable. If you focus only on physical symptoms and hold the belief that those symptoms are only treatable with modern medicine, you will find recurrence of symptoms, development of chronic symptoms, and worsening physical conditions because the mind, body, and energy influence each other. Prana, the vital life-force energy, is an essential factor in your well-being, and yoga and Ayurveda help you understand, move, and work with prana.

Working with prana helps you in the moment and also as you age. As the years pass, you don't have to fall apart in painful ways, piece by piece. You can take care of yourself by nourishing all parts of you (mind, body, and spirit), and age more gracefully and easefully. To be able to do that, it will help you to understand prana.

The vital life-force energy, prana, is the ¹
The natural and whole foods you eat cont⁻
the exercise and rest you take helps pr
help you consciously move life-force

QUOTE

Prana gives emotional harmony, balanc
—Dr. David Frawley, author of *Yoga and A*
Self-Realization

How to Assist the Flow of Prana

Prana is considered the subtle essence of vata, and when vata
of balance it affects the flow of prana in the body. One of the best ways
calm vata and help prana flow through the body is with yogic breathing, or
pranayama. You'll notice that in yoga classes, pranayama (breath control)
is an essential component, and that's because your breath is directly related
to prana. By directing your breath, you direct your energy (prana), which
boosts your stamina, energy, and focus. That flow of energy recharges your
mind and body.

TWO SIMPLE WAYS TO FEEL PRANA

1. Notice how you feel mentally, emotionally, and physically before your
   yoga practice or before a nice, brisk walk outside. Then, after your practice (or your walk), take some time to notice any changes you feel in
   your mood or in your body. If you are feeling more balanced, more centered, and happier in mind and body, you're noticing the effect of prana
   flowing through the body and nourishing the cells.
2. Rub your hands together vigorously and breathe in and out three times,
   slowly. Gently separate your hands to create a small space between your
   palms. You will begin to feel sensation and pulsing in your hands. This is
   the sensation of prana moving.

o Recognize Vata Imbalance

When any of the doshas are acting in excess in the body, you can notice this from how you're feeling mentally, emotionally, and physically. If you notice the early signs of imbalance, then you can start to create balance before symptoms get worse and disease follows. There are some very clear signs of vata imbalance that you can look for.

Physical Symptoms of Excess Vata

Vata moves throughout the body and affects the bones and the colon in particular. Because vata's elements are air and space, when you want to remember the signs of vata imbalance, think of the qualities that go with air and space, such as cool, dry, light, and mobile. Keeping in mind those qualities, it makes sense that the following are some ways you can tell if you are experiencing excess vata.

EARLY PHYSICAL SIGNS OF VATA IMBALANCE

- Dry mouth and dry skin
- Constipation
- Short and shallow breathing
- Cold hands and feet
- Inability to sit still and focus
- Excess gas: burping, hiccoughs, etc.
- Insomnia

When you notice these early signs, you can take action by your choice of foods, routine, etc., to help balance vata and begin to create balance and health again. You could start by making sure your diet is vata pacifying by eating at regular times and by giving yourself an oil massage at least once per day with sesame oil or specially prepared herbalized oil for vata. If you're experiencing constipation, your specialist will likely recommend you take the herb triphala, as well.

Emotional and Mental Signs of Vata Imbalance

When vata is in excess, it affects your mental clarity and your emotional balance. There are easy ways to tell if vata is influencing your state of mind.

MENTAL SIGNS OF VATA IMBALANCE

- Anxiety
- Fear
- Whirling, crowded, and continual stream of thoughts
- Disturbed sleep

When you experience these symptoms, even though they are *mental* symptoms, you can ameliorate them with *physical* practices. So, for example, drinking hot water with lemon, making sure you're eating enough at meals, having some warm milk before bed, practicing vata-pacifying pranayama, and other such actions will help with your mental state.

ESSENTIAL

Your Ayurvedic specialist may suggest an enema if you are experiencing symptoms of excess vata. An enema is a way to purify the body, and under guidance or by the suggestion of your specialist, it can be an effective way to treat vata disorders.

When vata imbalance continues in the body, it can lead to certain types of arthritis, more serious digestive disorders, chronic lower back pain, and emotional imbalances. So, if you catch the signs of vata imbalance early (for example, when you're experiencing anxiety or constipation), you can use Ayurveda as preventive care.

Practice Noticing Vata

Becoming aware of how vata is showing up in you can take a little bit of practice. You can start to notice how you are doing by taking time throughout the day to pause and notice.

Taking a Moment to Stop

Here's a simple exercise for you to try. Take time during the day to stop what you're doing, and just take a few moments to notice how you are. Do this daily to check in with yourself.

DAILY FIVE-MINUTE CHECK-IN

1. Log off of the computer.
2. Turn off your cell phone.
3. Sit down, and sit up straight. Place your feet firmly on the floor. Roll your shoulders up, back, and down.
4. Close your eyes.
5. Notice your breath. Is it shallow, short, long, deep? Watch the breath without changing it.
6. After you notice your breath, focus lightly on it.
7. Notice the mind's activity for several breaths. As thoughts come up, allow them to float by. Return your focus lightly to the breath so you don't get caught up in your mind's activity.
8. After watching the thoughts for several breaths, take a nice deep inhale and let it out on a longer exhale.
9. Return to normal breathing, and reflect on how your thoughts were: nervous, anxious, spinning, foggy, clear, optimistic?

If after this exercise, you notice that you experienced a lot of anxiety, fear, and worry, this is something to pay attention to. Everyone's mind will have thoughts during that type of meditation. It's natural for the mind to keep thinking. And you can pay attention to it and see if it's predominantly worried, foggy, or generally clear. If you notice you're experiencing anxiety and worry, try a vata-pacifying diet, plan some soothing activities, and hang out with supportive friends or family. And, most of all, do not judge yourself for having excess vata. With many to-dos and a culture that encourages fast-paced living and fast-paced eating, it's no wonder you may have excess vata. Have compassion for yourself.

Look Back on Your Day

Take some time at the end of the day to remember what you've done and how you've felt. Write down the following questions on a piece of paper, one at a time, and answer them:

1. What did I do right after I woke up this morning?
2. How was I feeling when I woke up this morning?
3. Was I rushing around this morning, running late, or wondering how I'd be able to squeeze everything into the day?
4. Did I make time to eat? How many meals? How did I feel when eating?
5. Did I find time for myself to take a pause, breathe, or laugh?
6. How am I feeling right now?

If you find that the answers to your questions have words that show you are anxious, getting overwhelmed, feeling spacey, and not taking time to pause or slow down, you may be aggravating vata or experiencing excess vata. It's very common in our modern world, with all the emphasis on movement, change, and multitasking, to create vata imbalance in the body. So, just notice, and then you can make some choices to balance vata.

Vata Time of Day, Year, and Life

Ayurveda views the body as a microcosm of the universe, and the body is affected by the changes and variations outside. There is a time of day, a time of year, and a time of life that is characterized as vata, which means your body will be experiencing the effects of the qualities of vata most at those times.

Calming Activities to Prepare for Vata Time

You'll notice the times of day have a cycle. The time between 2 P.M. and 6 P.M. and 2 A.M. to 6 A.M. is characterized by the qualities of vata. So, at these times of day, you are prone to experience more of vata's effects. Do you ever notice, for example, that if you wake up in the middle of the night from a racing mind, it's usually vata time?

I find it profound that Ayurveda provides us with contemplations within the twenty-four-hour day clock, within each passing season, and within the progression of our whole life. As a fall/winter (vata) constitution I feel extremely empowered knowing that during 2–6 a.m. and p.m. I need to be mindful of the rituals I enact to support myself.
—Danny Arguetty, author of *Nourishing the Teacher*

It's a great idea to do things during the afternoon hours to balance vata. So, for vata types, having a cup of decaffeinated hot tea or hot water with lemon between 2 and 6 P.M. is a better idea than having a cool ice cream bar. If the weather permits, take a nice, slow walk outside, and enjoy the afternoon's fresh air. Take long, deep breaths, and feel the grounding quality of the earth beneath your feet.

Even though 2–6 is vata time, to help balance excess vata it's important to create balance throughout the day, not just when those specific times occur. That's why it's helpful to do vata-pacifying routines in the morning, continue to eat vata-pacifying foods throughout your day, and nourish yourself with a gentle relaxation activity before bed.

ADHD shows up in adults and in children, and Ayurveda treats it as a vata imbalance. If your child has symptoms of ADHD, talk to your Ayurvedic specialist. She may recommend vata-pacifying activities and foods. Also, television and video games are stimulating for vata, so trade those activities for something calming, such as painting or drawing outside with sidewalk chalk.

Another great help for vata is to create routine. Try to make the mornings the same and predictable for yourself and your family. During the school week, have breakfast at the same time and have dinner at the same time each day when you can (around their extracurricular activities). Expect your children to go to bed at the same time each night (when possible), and have a bedtime routine. A bedtime routine for you (and your children) could look like this:

1. Turn off the television, computers, and cell phones an hour before bedtime.
2. Go outside for at least five minutes and get grounded and calm. Observe the moonlight, stars, and the nighttime sounds together. Everyone, take nice, soothing long breaths. Let go of the day.
3. Come inside, and slowly enjoy a cup of warm spiced milk.
4. Brush teeth and get dressed for bed, with as much calm and peacefulness as possible.
5. Get into bed, and before falling asleep enjoy sinking into the support of the bed. Take a few breaths, let go of the day even more, and think of at least one thing you're grateful for.

Having a nighttime routine will help you stay mindful of the transition from activity to sleep and can help children and adults alike feel secure and grounded.

During the Vata Times of Year

The vata time of year is considered fall/wintertime. It is the time of year characterized by dryness and cool temperatures. If your climate doesn't get cool and dry, then the "vata" time of year won't be something you need to balance. For the other places, though, it's important at this time of year to adjust your diet, make sure you wear warm clothes, take hot baths, drink hot liquids and soups, and do other such warming and moistening activities that your body and mind are asking for. Enjoy hot apple cider with cinnamon, and prepare your family's favorite grounding fall and winter stews. Allow the darkness of these months to tempt you to sink into cozy moments, under warm blankets, to relax and ground yourself.

Never Too Soon to Prepare for Vata Years

Vata time of life refers to your later years. That doesn't mean you should wait until those years to start taking care of vata imbalances. As soon as you can, keep an eye on vata imbalances. With a busy lifestyle, it's so easy for vata to become imbalanced at any age. And if you begin to take care of yourself and your family early on, it will set a good foundation for balancing your vata in later years, too.

Vata in Balance

When vata is in balance, the light, mobile, and expansive qualities of vata work to your advantage. Vata is necessary for your physical and mental functioning, and it helps you see things from a broad perspective. The qualities of vata, with prana as the subtle force, connect you to the energy that makes possible all movement and life.

Vata and a Sense of Security

When vata is in balance, you experience mental and emotional harmony. Vata in balance gives you the ability to think with agility, creativity, flexibility, and enthusiasm. When vata is in balance, your stable emotions and your ability to think clearly and efficiently give you a sense of well-being.

ESSENTIAL

Feeling secure, safe, and calm is important for vata types. If you experience excess vata and it's difficult for you to feel safe, the first step is to realize you can do things to counteract that feeling. The vata-pacifying yoga and breathing routines, food choices, and other tips (such as surrounding yourself with supportive people) can really help.

With vata in balance, you will feel more secure and stable because you are able to handle life well and from a grounded place: your emotions and fears aren't running the show.

Get Uplifted by Literature and the Arts

With vata in balance, you are also able to see the bigger picture of life: you are able to see the world around you as beautiful, and you can cultivate trust in the basic goodness of the universe. If you have trouble believing in the basic goodness of the universe, find authors, poets, and teachers whose writing gives you hope and faith that you are whole, that you are supported in the world, and that all is okay.

Finding supportive books will help you feel inspired about yourself and about the world around you. Carve out time in your life to read things that uplift you, or make it a habit to go to museums if art lights you up! Nourish your heart and mind with what others have taken time to create, and you may find kindred spirits through the ages through their work.

You digest what you experience in the world, just like you digest food. What choices you make for how to spend your time, what to read, and what to listen to affect your mental and physical well-being. You assimilate what your senses perceive, so seek out new ways to be with what's positive, inspiring, and imaginative in life.

While not all authors or teachers will appeal to you, there are so many voices out there that might strike a chord within you and help you feel supported and understood. Shop around and browse various books or art exhibits until you find what speaks to you. There is such variety when you consider even these works: the whimsically illustrated and supportive teachings of SARK (Susan Ariel Rainbow Kennedy), the Buddhist-inspired words of Pema Chödrön, the poetry of Rainer Maria Rilke, or—if you love visual art—the paintings of Wassily Kandinsky. (See the list of additional resources at the end of this book for suggestions.)

Color is the key. The eye is the hammer. The soul is the piano with its many chords. The artist is the hand that, by touching this or that key, sets the soul vibrating automatically. —Wassily Kandinsky

Choosing calming, inspiring, and supportive books and art supports vata in balance, which will lead you to feel balance, joy, and creative inspiration.

Physical Benefits of Vata in Balance

When vata is in balance it's easier to be in the present moment. At those times you can just be who you are, whether with others or alone. You can be present to what is, in a centered way, without worrying about what you should be doing, without needing to hurry to another activity, and without pressuring yourself to do the impossible. At these times, your body is in a relaxed state, your breath is regulated and steady, and your body is performing its vital functions with ease. When vata is in balance, your heart, digestion, and elimination are all being supported in a balanced, easeful way.

Strengthen Relationships by Recognizing Vata Imbalance

Most people are in relationship with others—dear friends, blood relatives, community, or partners. While it's *not* a good practice to walk around diagnosing other people just from your interactions with them, when it comes to those you live with or are very close to, it can be wonderful for your relationships if you can recognize a possible vata imbalance. Without mentioning anything to the person, you can simply be more mindful of how you interact with her at those times. This awareness can help your relationship become stronger.

When a Loved One Has Excess Vata

If you notice a loved one, including your child, is showing signs of excess vata—mental spaciness, inability to focus or sit still, dry skin, gas, anxiety, difficulty sleeping, etc.—you should make sure that you are not aggravating that condition. To do this, talk gently and slowly when you talk to him. Listen attentively when he talks; don't interrupt. See if you can make your energy calm, peaceful, and relaxed. If you often eat together or prepare meals for him, see if you can eat at regular times, slowly, and with mild, easy conversation. The environment you and your loved ones create will make a huge difference.

Telling Others If You're Feeling Imbalanced

You don't have to mention the word *vata* to your close friends who don't know Ayurveda, and still you can let them know that you're feeling anxious or insecure or needing support. That's what good friends are really for. And if you don't tell them how you are feeling, they won't know. The benefit for you is, if you tell them you are feeling anxious or worried, then perhaps they will be sensitive during your conversations or offer to listen or help. This is a wonderful support for a vata imbalance—loved ones being there to help you feel secure and safe. Keep in mind, people can't always tell what you're experiencing inside, especially if you're good at hiding it. So with those whom you feel safe around, let them in. Let them help you feel safe.

CHAPTER 8

How to Pacify Vata

When vata dosha is out of balance, there are several ways to pacify and soothe vata. Vata's qualities are dryness, mobility, and spaciousness, and when out of balance, vata dosha can cause you to feel cold, anxious, and spacey. So, to pacify vata, you'll treat yourself to experiences that have the opposite qualities. Also, if you know you have a predominance of vata dosha in your constitution, you can keep it in check before it becomes noticeably out of balance.

Keeping Vata in Balance

If you can keep vata pacified without waiting to see signs of imbalance, that is best. If you know you have a lot of vata in your constitution, then it won't be a surprise to you that during certain times of day, certain times of year, and later in life, you will need to be especially conscious of vata dosha.

Use Preventive Measures

Because you know what times of day, what times of year, and what times of life are considered vata times, you can take caution to be particularly nurturing during those times. Since vata time of day is 2–6 P.M. (and 2–6 A.M.), do your best to avoid activities that can make you stirred up or anxious during those hours. Try breathwork and yoga for vata at that time of day. Or soak in a hot bath, give yourself a soothing massage, or take a nap. You don't have to spend the whole four hours from 2–6 P.M. doing very soothing things, but try to do something calming for vata during those hours each day. Be mindful during vata time of day, and take breaks when you can.

ESSENTIAL

Talk to your Ayurvedic specialist about herbs for vata time of year if you are prone to vata imbalance. She may recommend you take ashwaganda, which can address some vata disorders, including joint discomfort and anxiety. Talk to your specialist about dosage and if it would be right for you, any time of year, and particularly during vata season.

Because the fall and winter are vata times of year and your later years of life are vata years, these are times in your life to be particularly aware of how you are affected. Do what you can to stay warm: drink plenty of warm liquids, give yourself warm oil massages at least once per day, eat warm foods, and calm your mind. The darkness of the wintertime can aid meditation and introspection, so use that to your advantage. Calming the mind and warming the body are especially important during vata season and vata time of life. Because you know this, you can start taking care of vata before you notice particular imbalances.

Enjoy the Benefits of Vata

It's very important to keep an eye on yourself to see if vata is out of balance. It's also important to be grateful for the wonderful aspects of vata—all of the bodily functions it assists (including the workings of the heart and circulatory system) and how it helps the mind and your connection to higher levels of consciousness. So take time, while being careful to balance vata, to also appreciate it for all it offers with its movement, expansiveness, and airy qualities.

Great Foods for Vata

As always with the doshas, remember that like increases like and opposites balance. So you'll need to remember the qualities that are associated with vata and then choose foods that have the opposite qualities. Vata qualities are dry, airy, and cool, so you'll choose foods that are moist, dense, and warm. Also, when you eat, take time to sit down and eat slowly. Savor the tastes, aromas, and textures. Don't talk too much, watch TV, or read while eating. Focus just on eating, and relax.

Whole Grains and Protein for Vata

According to Dr. Lad, for vata it's best to have about 50 percent of your diet be whole grains. Have 20 percent protein, 20 to 30 percent vegetables, and an optional 10 percent fruit. (For vatas, remember it's best to cook the fruit and vegetables and add warming spices for taste and to enhance digestion.)

The best whole grains for vata are cooked oats, quinoa, and rice. Again, remember that you want to avoid dry foods, so even though rice is a wonderful grain for vata, rice cakes are not.

Legumes are a great source of protein. Examples of legumes for vata include lentils, mung beans, mung dahl, and occasionally tofu. Tofu is processed, so it's best to have it in moderation.

Many proteins are just fine for vata: beef, chicken, salmon, sardines, seafood, and tuna are all nourishing for someone of vata constitution.

Fruits and Vegetables for Vata

One of the qualities of vata is cold, so choose to eat foods that are warm in temperature and/or in their energetic qualities. Some warming foods that are great for vata are sweet fruits (not dried), such as apples (cooked), coconut, grapes, oranges, peaches, and strawberries. Vegetables should be cooked, and most vegetables would be great for vata when cooked, including asparagus, carrots, leafy greens, sweet potatoes, spaghetti squash, spinach, and zucchini.

Nuts, Seeds, and Condiments

For vata, nuts and seeds are great. It's best to eat them in moderation, and soak almonds in water overnight to make them easier to digest. Some examples of nuts to enjoy are almonds, cashews, pecans, peanuts, pine nuts, pistachios, and walnuts.

ESSENTIAL

When it comes to popcorn, eat it in moderation and add condiments to it to balance its airy qualities. Popcorn isn't a great snack choice for vata. If you are going to eat popcorn, you could add ghee or olive oil to it to balance the dry and airy qualities. Salt and pepper are fine for vata, too.

Seeds to add to your meals include chia, flax, halva, pumpkin, and sesame. You can add them on top of your cooked vegetables or your grains to add texture and essential nutrients.

Most condiments are fine for vata, but just remember that in your diet you want to cut down on processed foods. So, if you want pickled relish, choose the most natural ingredients in that relish, and the same goes for ketchup. Great ideas for condiments for vata constitution are gomasio, kelp, kombu, salt, seaweed, and tamari.

Aromas to Calm Vata

Aromas are helpful tools for balancing the doshas. Aromas are apparent in foods, herbs, and spices, as well as in essential oils. You can be intentional about the aromas you're cooking with. And because a warm bath is balancing for vata dosha, if you have a predominance of vata in your constitution, you would benefit from a soothing warm bath with aromatherapy. Self-massage is also a grounding practice for vata, and you can mix massage oil with soothing aromas for vata.

Aromas in Foods for Vata

Experiment with aromas and see which ones work best for you. In general, cooking with cardamom, cinnamon, ginger, nutmeg, and clove could be beneficial to vata. Each time you make yourself a meal, remember this is a chance to fill your kitchen with aromas. For example, if you're in the mood for an apple, cook the apple in honey, and don't forget to sprinkle it with at least one spice, such as cinnamon. Experiment with the various aromas, learning which scents affect you in positive ways. Don't be afraid to get creative and try combinations that you've never tried before.

Aromas for the Bath or Massage Oil for Vata

Essential oils are not meant to be put directly onto the skin. You can mix essential oils in high-quality oil, such as extra-virgin, cold-pressed olive oil or sesame oil, and then put a few drops of that mixture into your bath or onto your skin. The typical way to figure out the ratio of base oil to essential oil is to measure the base oil in milliliters, then divide that number in half. That number is the maximum number of drops of essential oil you'll need to add to the mix. It doesn't take much; essential oils are very potent.

Aromas that are balancing for vata are pine, lavender, and frankincense. Try them out for yourself, and see which ones work best for you. Since everyone is unique, you will have your preference. Red rose, musk, and camphor, because of their sweet and warming tones, can also balance vata.

Routine for Vata

Keeping to a daily routine will help vata. Routine creates a structure that can help ground and stabilize the vata energy. If a vata type knows she has a schedule, it's easier for her to focus and stay on task. When the options get too numerous, a vata type could find herself feeling indecisive and unable to focus on any one thing.

Morning Routine

For vata, doing the morning routine slowly and mindfully is key. Wake up around 6 or 7 A.M., and know that you have an hour to do your morning rituals. Take your time cleaning your teeth, gums, tongue, eyes, ears, nose, and mouth. Choose to do breathwork and yoga postures that are soothing, grounding, calming, and stabilizing. Drink warm water, and take a warm bath or shower. Transition mindfully into your waking hours.

FACT

Vata types are prone to having difficulty falling asleep and staying asleep. If you're a vata type, you may wake up in the middle of the night between 2 and 6 A.M.: vata time. So your morning and evening routines are particularly important to calm and ground your mobile and potentially anxious energy.

After you've done your morning routine, have a warm and soothing breakfast. Take your time eating, and if you can, eat breakfast in silence. Sit down, and focus just on your morning meal. Enjoy the warmth and nourishing qualities of your breakfast.

Daytime Routine

For vata, it will help if you eat lunch at the same time every day. It matters less what exact time it is and more that you do it around the same time each day. Ideally, start eating between 11 A.M. and noon. Relax, chew your food slowly, and don't talk too much while eating. In the afternoon, when the clock strikes 2 P.M., be mindful that you're headed into vata time. Take care of yourself from 2–6 P.M., knowing this is the time that vata could become heightened. Take some breaks from work if you can. Take a tea break, find time for a nap, or take a walk outside and feel the grounding energy of the earth. Here is a standing meditation you can do at any time of day to help you feel grounded.

STANDING MEDITATION

1. Stand with feet parallel, hip-width apart.
2. Spread the toes and press evenly and firmly down through the four corners of each foot.
3. Release the tailbone down while lifting the sternum and crown of the head up. Stand tall with the arms by the sides, shoulders relaxed.
4. Relax the muscles in the face, shoulders, and belly.
5. Seal the lips and begin to breathe, slowly and steadily, through the nostrils. Draw deep breaths in and out.
6. With your feet hip-width apart, turn the toes in and heels out just a bit, so the feet are slightly pigeon-toed.
7. Exhale and bend the knees slightly. Let the shin bones move forward and then drop down into the force of gravity. Balance the weight evenly on the heels and balls of the feet and then let them sink into the earth.
8. Soften the gaze. Place both hands on the belly, and relax the belly and all of its contents.
9. Relax the muscles in the thighs and buttocks. Use as little muscular effort as possible. Let the bones support you. Feel the bones becoming heavy and surrender their weight to gravity.
10. Let yourself sink into the stance. Soften the muscles in the legs and sink into the support of the bones. Allow yourself to connect to the strength and support they have to offer.

11. To release, bring the feet back to parallel, inhale, and sweep the arms to the sides and overhead as the legs straighten. Press the palms together and exhale them down to prayer position at the heart. Take a deep breath in and let out an audible sigh.

Pause and feel the echo of the meditation in the mind and body, tuning in to what is present. Enjoy this standing meditation anytime you need to experience grounding and stability in your life.

Evening Routine for Vata

It's very important for vata types to eat dinner mindfully and slowly. Eating around 6 P.M. would be ideal. If you were to eat dinner around 6 P.M., it would be fine to continue to do some work for about an hour after dinner. Stopping stimulating activity by 8:30 P.M. would be really supportive for vata. At that point, do some calming and soothing activities with your family, friends, or by yourself. Let the mind relax. Spend time feeling nurtured and grounded. Around 9 P.M., start an evening self-care routine to get ready for bed.

ESSENTIAL

Drinking a cup of warm milk before bed has soothing qualities for vata constitution. You can add a teaspoon of ghee and a few spices, such as turmeric, cardamom, and cinnamon or nutmeg, for enhanced vata-balancing qualities. Ghee is a wonderful antidote for vata's dry and brittle qualities.

Before going to bed, it's great for vata to do a self-massage, particularly of the feet and the crown of the head. Take your time massaging the feet with warm oil, and luxuriate in the sensations as you massage your feet. Take nice, deep breaths. After massaging your feet, wash your hands with warm, soapy water, and then apply oil to the crown of your head and forehead. This type of massage is very soothing and calming for vata.

Try to get into bed by 10 P.M. Have enough blankets to keep yourself warm. You may find you'll sleep well with heavy blankets, as the weight of the blankets feels grounding and secure. Do what you can to feel warm and grounded.

Breathwork for Vata

Sudha Carolyn Lundeen, RN, Ayurvedic health and lifestyle coach, and 200- and 500-hour yoga teacher-trainer at Kripalu Center, in Lenox, Massachusetts designed the following breathwork section and yoga sequence for vata types. Contact her at *www.sudhalundeen.com* to order her *Taming the Winds of Vata* CD, which guides you through another yoga sequence for balancing vata dosha.

The purity of the air you breathe is, of course, very important. But how you breathe is equally if not more important—at the cellular level and as it impacts your thoughts and feelings. When vata dosha goes out of balance, you may feel a heightened sense of indecisiveness, anxiety, and fear. Anxiety and fear tend to affect the breath by producing short, shallow upper-chest breathing. Thus, the most important breathing practices to tame vata dosha are those that produce a calm and steady breath pattern.

Nadi Shodhana

One of the most well-known breathing techniques for producing a calm and steady breath pattern is **nadi shodhana**, an alternate nostril, channel purifying, and balancing breath. To do this, breathe in through one nostril, and exhale out the other. Then, inhale through that side and exhale out the first.

Understanding the Nadis

When speaking of the power of the breath, it's helpful to know about the nadi system. **Nadis** are the energy channels of the body that provide the "vehicle" for the flow of prana (life force) and consciousness throughout the entire body. The central nadi is called the **Sushumna**, which runs from the base or root of the spinal column (muladhara chakra) to the crown of the head (sahasrara chakra). Two other important nadis, the Ida and Pingala begin at the base of the spine, crisscross over and around the Sushumna, and end up together at the crown of the head. The **chakras** are energy vortexes (sometimes described as spinning wheels of energy) that exist where the Ida and Pingala cross.

The Ida ends at the left hemisphere of the brain (some say the left nostril), and the Pingala ends at the right. The Ida has cooling properties and relates to the feminine principle. The Pingala has heating properties and relates to the masculine principle.

ESSENTIAL

Throughout the day the breath automatically fluctuates between the two nadis. There is a shift from right to left nostrils being open about every sixty to ninety minutes in the healthy person. This balancing of Ida and Pingala causes prana to flow evenly and is part of the natural balancing process of the body.

When the nadis are clear and balanced, certain external signs appear. They are lightness and leanness of the body, brilliancy in complexion, increased gastric fire, and the absence of restlessness in the body. These are some obvious signs of a healthy body.

INSTRUCTIONS FOR NADI SHODHANA

1. Sit comfortably with the spine straight.
2. Hold your right hand in Vishnu mudra (the hand position where the thumb, ring finger, and pinky are extended, and the other fingers are bent).
3. Close off the right nostril with the right thumb.
4. Softly breathe in through the left nostril.
5. At the top of that breath, close off the left nostril with the right ring finger and exhale through the right nostril.
6. At the bottom of that exhale, breathe back in the right nostril.
7. At the top of that inhale, close off the right nostril with the right thumb and exhale out the left nostril.
8. Repeat this pattern for a minute or two, keeping the breath soft, regular, and steady, and the shoulders relaxed.

If your arm gets tired, you can prop it on a cushion or with your other hand. When the nadis are open, there is a natural feeling of calm and ease of being.

QUESTION

Do I have to use the Vishnu mudra hand position?
You may use Vishnu mudra or the power of the mind to imagine one nostril opening and the other closing. By focusing attention on the closed or less open nostril, it will gradually open. This can take a while to master, but with practice, it will happen.

Dirgha Breath

Another important breath is **Dirgha** breath, the three-part or yogic breath. When you do this, you welcome the breath deep into the lungs, causing the belly and ribs to expand three-dimensionally. An easy way to learn this is by lying on your back with the knees bent. Once in this position, follow these instructions:

DIRGHA BREATH, LYING ON YOUR BACK

1. Place your hands on the belly, pressing down slightly to give a bit of resistance as you breathe in.
2. Inhale deeply so that the hands rise as you breathe in.
3. Simply relax and exhale. Practice this a while. Then rest.
4. Place your hands over the sides of your ribs. As you breathe in, try to make your ribs expand outward into your hands. Imagine your sides having fish gills as you breathe through them.
5. Place one hand on the upper chest and collarbones and the other on the back side of your shoulders, just below the neck. As you inhale, try to breathe so deeply that even these two areas expand.
6. Combine all three aspects of this breath. Breathing in, belly, side ribs, and upper chest and back expand with the movement of the breath flowing into the lungs. Breathing out, empty out. Release and let go.

Practice Dirgha breath for one to five minutes. Then pause and notice the effect. You will likely feel calmer and more grounded, awake and clear. That is, you will feel more "balanced." A major goal of Ayurveda is achieving that sense of a balanced state in body and mind.

Warming Breath

The warming breath helps correct the cooling tendency of vata. The right nostril relates to the Pingala, or Sun energy, side. Using the same hand position as in nadi shodhana, start by breathing in the right nostril and exhaling out the left. Repeat. Breathe back in the right and breathe out the left. Continue for a minute or so.

So Hum Steady Breath

This is a steady in-and-out breath, combined with the silent repetition of the words (mantra) *So* and *Hum*. The breath naturally makes these two sounds: *Sooooooo* as you inhale and *Hummmmmm* as you exhale. This practice is very helpful in balancing the Ida and Pingala.

1. Place your hands over your ears, and as you breathe in, silently say the word *so*. Let the "soooo" extend the full length of the in-breath.
2. As you breathe out, silently say the word *hum*, extending that sound for the full length of the exhalation.

Once you get the gist of this, continue the practice with your hands resting comfortably in your lap. And, remember, for all of these breathing practices, it is important to be seated comfortably, head aligned over the spine, with your back upright and shoulders relaxed.

Yoga Practice for Vata Management

When thinking about your yoga practice, remember that vata dosha is associated with the elements space and air. The key qualities of these elements are cold, light, dry, rough, and mobile. Vata dosha will become imbalanced if your activities and other lifestyle choices increase those qualities. The route to bringing vata back to balance is to favor activities that are calming and grounding. A regular yoga, meditation, and breathing practice can do wonders, in conjunction with the vata-pacifying lifestyle choices you make off your yoga mat.

Although it's true that each pose has specific effects on the doshas, when considering which postures to practice, remember that how you practice the pose is more important than which pose you choose.

TIPS FOR A VATA-PACIFYING YOGA PRACTICE

- Practice in a quiet, grounded, and systematic way.
- Stay warm; wear layers.
- Pay attention to all of your joints. Begin your practice with gentle circling of the joints—this gets them warmed up, and they will become naturally lubricated for subsequent movements.
- Aim to work on strength, stamina, and flexibility. Too much of any one of those is its own kind of imbalance.
- Strengthen the core, and hold poses a little longer than you are inclined to. Practice being present; calm the mind by focusing on sensation and breath.
- Keep poses condensed rather than expansive. Practice drawing energy downward from the head into the belly and legs.
- Move from your core; connect to your bones. Keep the four corners of each foot "rooted" into the floor (especially the base of the big toe).

Most poses are good for balancing vata. Some are more inherently calming and grounding. As vata "resides" in the large intestine, pelvic area, and lower abdomen, poses that compress or stretch these areas will help balance vata.

Poses to be avoided or modified are those that are overly stimulating to the nervous system, such as rapid vinyasa sequences or postures that put excessive pressure on the joints—especially the neck, shoulders, and knees.

Standing Yoga Poses

Standing poses strengthen the body, steady the mind, and build concentration. After doing gentle joint warm-ups, do one or more of the following standing postures.

TADASANA: MOUNTAIN POSE

1. Stand with your feet hip-width distance apart. Feel your feet, especially the base of the big toe, firmly planted on the ground.
2. Engage the legs, tuck your tailbone under slightly, and lift up through the crown of your head.
3. Inhale and lift the shoulders up.
4. Exhale and roll the shoulders back and down.
5. Inhale. On the exhale, with your arms by your sides, extend the fingers so that the fingertips point toward the earth. Feel the downward energy grounding you.
6. Take nice, long, deep breaths in and out as you gently fix your gaze out in front of you.
7. Envision yourself tall, strong, and heavy like a mountain—grounded in the earth and majestically connected to the sky. Keep breathing.
8. After several breaths in Mountain Pose, stay standing and relax the posture. Notice how you feel.

UTKATASANA: CHAIR POSE

1. While standing with feet hip-width distance apart, feel your feet firmly rooted on the earth, and inhale.
2. As you exhale, pull the belly button toward the spine, engaging the abdomen. Soften the knees and pretend to sit down into an imaginary chair. Fire up the leg muscles. Relax the shoulders. Breathe rhythmically in and out.
3. On exhale, raise your arms out in front of you, shoulder height and parallel to the earth. Softly gaze in front of you. If you feel any strain in the lower back or knees, lower the arms, engage the abdominals more firmly, or simply come out of the pose.
4. Hold this posture for three to five breaths. As you hold the posture, be curious about the effects of the pose. Notice sensations such as heat rising or that you're feeling more connected to the earth. Release the pose by pressing your feet into the earth, standing up tall, and releasing the arms to the sides of your body.
5. From time to time, hold the posture for one breath longer than you think you can, gently challenging your beliefs and deepening your practice.

VIRABHADRASANA, WARRIOR I

1. Start by standing in Tadasana, Mountain Pose, with your feet hip-width apart and firmly pressing into the floor.
2. Place your hands on your hips and inhale. On the exhale, take a big step back with your left foot, keeping both feet pointing forward.
3. Press the base of the big and little toes of the front foot firmly into the floor. The heel of the back foot should press toward the floor. For greater stability, place a rolled towel or small cushion under the back heel. Align your hips so they face directly forward.
4. Keeping a strong abdominal core, lift the arms out to the sides and overhead in a "V" position, palms facing each other.
5. Continue to breathe with a steady inhale and exhale. Maintain a soft gaze on one spot. Imagine yourself a warrior: impressively strong and focused. Feel the heat rising as you hold the posture, and feel the earth supporting you.
6. To release this posture, lower the arms to your sides or hips, and on the exhale step the back foot up to meet the front.
7. Repeat the Warrior Pose, this time taking a big step back with the right foot.

TREE POSE

1. Stand in Tadasana, feet hip-width apart and firmly pressing into the floor.
2. Shift your weight onto the left foot.
3. Bring the sole of the right foot to rest on the inner ankle of the left foot. The knee should point outward. Stabilize yourself; feel balanced.
4. Slide the right foot up the leg (pausing at the knee or upper inner thigh). Press your foot and leg into each other for better balance.
5. Fix your gaze on a steady point in front of you. Maintain a steady, soft gaze. Keep the breath steady and slow.
6. When you feel stable, raise the arms into a "V" position overhead and relax the shoulders.
7. Imagine yourself being a tree that can bend in the wind, while remaining stable and solid.
8. Hold this posture for a few more breaths, focusing the gaze and the mind.

9. To release this posture, exhale the arms down to your sides. Lower the right foot to the ground.
10. Repeat this posture on the other side.

Yoga poses on the floor help ground energy, build strength, and increase flexibility.

NAVASANA, BOAT POSE, BELLY DOWN

1. Lie on the ground, belly down, arms at your sides.
2. Place your forehead or chin on the floor. Press your pubic bone into the floor.
3. Reach both feet toward the back of the room so that both legs are slightly off the ground. Hold for a few breaths.
4. Release the posture, turn your head to one side, and relax.
5. Bring your forehead or chin to the floor. Inhale. On exhale, press your pubic bone into the earth. Reach your feet toward the back of the room so that both legs are straight and slightly lifted off the ground.
6. Try to touch the back wall with your fingers, arms lifting off the floor, aligned with the torso. Take a few more breaths. See if you can lift your arms and legs a bit higher. Notice how they become more or less willing and how they change with repetitions. Continue to breathe.
7. To release, lower your legs and arms, turning your head to the side. Take a few breaths.

GARBASANA, CHILD POSE

1. Come into Table Pose. From Navasana, draw your hands underneath your shoulders, press up into the position so that your arms are straight, with your shoulders lined up over your wrists. Keep your knees on the floor, bent at 90-degree angles, with the hips aligned over the knees.
2. With knees either together or apart, lower your hips onto your heels. (If your sitting bones don't reach your heels, put a small cushion on top of your heels so your sitting bones can rest on that cushion.)
3. Keep your hands on the floor, arms stretched out over your head, as you place your forehead on the earth. Feel the earth supporting you at all

the points where you're touching the ground. (If your forehead doesn't touch the earth, you can prop your forehead up with your hands, or use a cushion here, too.)

4. Take some long, deep breaths, so deep it might feel like you are filling the lower back and lungs with air. Take several steady breaths.
5. To release this posture, come up to hands and knees, and then lie down on your right side in fetal position to rest.

SHAVASANA, REST POSE

1. Come into a position lying on your back with legs, torso, and shoulders aligned.
2. If you wish, to ease tension in the back, you can place a bolster or cushion under your knees.
3. Cover yourself with blankets to stay warm.
4. Cover your eyes with an eye pillow or scarf to block out light and quiet the mind.
5. Let yourself melt down into the support of the earth.
6. Lie in Rest Pose. Let go of all "doing." Relax.
7. When you're ready to come out of the pose, roll over onto your right side into a fetal position. Then, press up into a seated posture. Take a moment to give thanks for some of the gifts in your life. Move into the rest of your day with grace and ease.

Keep in mind that for vata, regularity, rhythm, and consistency of practice are key. Vata types tend to want to jump around and keep trying out new things. See if you can stick with these postures, and notice their effects before following the urge to move on to something else.

Consult with your doctors and healers before doing yoga. During practice, if you feel any sharp pain, stop what you're doing and relax. Consult your doctor before taking on any new physical practice like yoga, especially if you are pregnant or have cardiovascular or respiratory conditions.

CHAPTER 9

Understanding Pitta

Pitta is the only dosha of the three with fire in it, so it's precious for that hot quality. Pitta's heat supports so much in the body, especially in the way of digestion, transformation, and vitality. Heat supports the sharpness of the mind and passion of the heart. Pitta types have a lot to offer the world with their ability to get things done and blaze new trails. It's very important, as it is with all of the doshas, to keep pitta in balance so its wonderful qualities support your healthy living.

What Is Pitta?

Pitta dosha is of the elements fire and water. The fiery qualities of pitta mean that a predominantly pitta-type person normally has good digestion and a good deal of willpower, passion, and determination to get things done. Pitta's qualities include liquid, oily, hot, light, fluid, and intense.

Strong Momentum of Pitta

Two of the qualities of pitta—fire and fluidity—help you come up with great ideas, accomplish goals, and push projects to completion. The sharpness of the pitta mind loves to achieve, and the fiery momentum helps burn through obstacles to that end.

QUESTION

What are the physical signs of a predominantly pitta person?
The physical attributes of pitta can be reddish hair or baldness; moderate body; freckles; sharp eyes that are brown, hazel, or green. Pittas are usually of moderate build. But remember you don't need to have all these qualities to have a good deal of pitta in your constitution. These are simple ways of viewing the likelihood of pitta being present.

It's very important for a pitta person who is on the move and on a mission (whether in business or with family) to keep her pitta balanced so she doesn't start to get too pushy, angry, annoyed, and judgmental. While it is exciting and creates a great sense of accomplishment to keep up the momentum and fuel the fire, it's important to balance that fire so others will enjoy working with you and supporting you as you reach your goals. You won't cool off too much if you balance your fire: you'll still shine, shine, shine, and you'll do it with more finesse and joy if you don't get yourself overheated.

Pitta's Subtle Energy: Tejas

The subtle force of pitta is tejas. It's important to keep tejas in balance, and the same methods for balancing pitta will work with tejas. So, at the basic level, it's good for you to know that, like the other doshas, pitta has a subtle energy at work. If you just keep in mind the doshas and working with them, it will help their subtle energies, as well.

To calm overstimulated tejas, as you would do with pitta, be mindful of your diet, your exercise, and the use of stimulants. When your fire is too hot, you want to cool it down to protect your immune system, your tissues, your organs, and your mind from burnout.

How to Recognize Pitta Imbalance

When you wonder about what excess pitta could look like for the mind and body, think about the effects of heat. Imagine what effects hot oil could have on the insides of your body (since pitta is hot and oily).

Hotheaded Pitta

A person who is hotheaded is known to be easily angered and can fly off the handle without much warning. To others, a hotheaded person's reactions can seem unfounded, unwarranted, and too much to handle. Too much pitta also affects the mind, causing it to experience jealousy and control issues, which can be detrimental to relationships in work and in the home. When pitta is in excess, you can become domineering and hard to please.

QUOTE

Pitta types lose control with great rapidity. It takes a great deal of awareness for them to remember that other humans—namely vata and kapha—inhabit the planet. —Maya Tiwari

If your pitta is out of control, it can be detrimental to relationships, and all that fire is a lot for your body and mind to experience. If you are predominantly pitta and your pitta is in excess, you may not realize that it's not healthy to be constantly hot, pushing, and exerting yourself. It does take a toll, over the long haul, on your health.

Also, if you are hard to please and controlling, it affects your ability to experience a deep sense of love, trust, and joy when in relationship (work or otherwise) with others. By balancing your pitta, you could open up to a more collaborative and harmonious existence in your work and home life . . . and still be outstandingly productive.

Volcanic Eruptions and the Physical Body

A good way to remember what effects pitta has on the physical body is to think of it as though there were molten lava in the body. Imagine how molten lava spurts and spreads from a volcano. So, when pitta is aggravated, it can lead to such things as acne, rash, ulcers, heartburn, loose stools, and excess urine. And due to pitta's spreading nature, one may find it spilling into other parts of the body, as well.

A Quiz about Your Pitta

It may be hard for you to recognize if your pitta is in excess, especially if you are used to living that way. Take a moment to answer these questions.

- Do you compare yourself to others, feeling competitive in nature?
- Are you often irritated with your family members or close friends?
- Do you look at what your colleagues or coworkers are doing and think of ways they could be doing their jobs better?
- Does it bother you if the books on your shelf aren't organized in exactly the way you think is best?
- Are you often sure that your way is the right way?

Be honest with yourself when you answer these questions. If you answer yes to many of them, you may want to really make sure that your pitta is in check. When pitta is in excess, it's one reason that pitta's life span tends to be moderately long rather than very long. They burn their energy so quickly that what they have will last fewer years. And you could be making the people around you more uncomfortable than you'd want to while also adding unnecessary stress to your own life. You are full of potential and brightness, so it can be a struggle to not overdo it.

Pitta in Balance

When pitta is in balance, you are a very bright light. You're sleeping well, your digestion is working well, and your mind is sharp and active. You are grounded and secure and able to accomplish things while also taking time off to relax, play, and be full of compassion.

By the Light of Your Fire

Pitta types shine in the world through their desire and ability to make things happen. Their enthusiasm for accomplishments and leading the way means they produce, create, and then share their final product and the knowledge they've gained. Pittas don't tend to work quietly at home and enjoy their success alone; they like to share their knowledge and expertise.

Pittas are smart and capable. They tend to be doctors, engineers, teachers, and lawyers. They also do well with public engagements because they are charismatic. Pittas may be drawn to become politicians, especially because they believe strongly in their principles and are drawn to leadership positions.

Even in a domestic sense, pittas will adhere to their principles. They will be happiest when they create order and are fastidious about cleanliness.

About Your Daily Habits

For pitta types, it's important that when you get hungry you eat, otherwise you can become irritable and experience hypoglycemia. Because you have a strong digestive fire, it's important to make sure you take time to eat three meals per day and be aware of which snacks are supportive to your type.

It's likely that you will prefer to stay up late—past midnight. You may find yourself wanting to read yourself to sleep, late at night. And that's okay, because your sleep will be sound and moderate in length. If you can, though, take a break between reading and sleeping to do a calming pranayama or visualization. This is because pitta's dreams can be tumultuous.

Pitta Time of Day, Year, and Life

As it is with all three doshas, pitta energy is the predominant force during certain times of day, times of year, and a time of life. When these times in nature are predominant, you can take advantage of pitta's qualities and also be careful not to exacerbate them.

The Heat of the Day

The pitta time of the day is 10 A.M.–2 P.M. This is the time when your body is doing its work for digestion. It's digesting what you're eating and what you're taking in with all your senses. It's a fiery time, so you can eat your largest meal at this time. Also, because it's a fiery time, try not to do strenuous activity or have sensitive conversations at this time of day. Keep your activities to a moderate, steady pace.

It's also pitta time from 10 P.M.–2 A.M. You'll likely be asleep during this time, and sleep is good for you during pitta time. At this time, while your senses are relaxed, your body can focus on digesting all the food and information you took in while you were awake.

Pitta Time of Year

Summertime is pitta time of year. That's why you'll dash to meet the ice cream truck, you'll pull out your swimsuit, and you'll take vacations to the beach. When you are drawn to play on the beach, try not to do it during the pitta time of day. If you do, be sure to cool yourself off before and after by drinking cool drinks, massaging yourself with coconut oil, sitting in the shade, and listening to soothing music on your iPod.

ACTIVITIES FOR THE SUMMER TO BALANCE PITTA

1. Play in sprinklers on the lawn.
2. Massage your whole body with coconut oil.
3. Swim in a lake, ocean, or pool.
4. Stay in during the hot hours of the day, and do something relaxing, such as reading a book or playing with arts and crafts.

5. Lie in a hammock underneath the shady trees.
6. At night, admire the stars and the moon, noticing the moon's cooling vibration.
7. Before getting into bed, practice shitali breath, to cool yourself down after a busy day.

Remembering to take extra care to cool yourself down during the summer months will help you keep your pitta in check. You'll feel healthier, happier, and more balanced if you continue to create balance for yourself in the heat.

Pitta Time of Life

Your pitta years are the middle years of your life. When you've become an adult and before you're in your wisest years, you are in your pitta years. During these years, you are experiencing the height of your energy to create, desirous to find out who you are and what your mark will be on the world. These are the years you are gaining knowledge, skills, and expertise, then putting it all to use. These are when you make adult friendships, create your own family and community, and begin to put your unique stamp on all that you do.

Enjoy these pitta years. Learn, experience, and find out who you uniquely are so you can share your particular gifts. And take time to balance your hard work with relaxation—get in some bodywork and spend time relaxing with friends or family.

When Your Children Are Heated Up

There's so much you can do for your children to keep their pitta in balance. If you have a child who is predominantly pitta, when you add things into his life to balance pitta's qualities he will be able to continue those practices when he is older (especially in the pitta time of his life).

You can disguise pitta-pacifying things as fun, cooling activities and special family-time excursions for you and your children.

For Your Achieving Child

Being able to get all As in school, play first base on the baseball team, and be the star in the school play every year is one way that pitta types may be able to gain supportive recognition. Bright and capable children will work hard, especially when they are encouraged and rewarded for their achievements. They may get rewards, such as getting into the best schools, attending the best universities, and getting jobs in fields they are passionate about. Working hard and gaining experience in leadership roles help the pitta child as life goes on, too. She may be the president of student council or the editor of the school magazine. Schools separate the "gifted and talented," and many schools will help the very bright, talented children to keep pushing themselves to their potential. (And hopefully the schools will help all students reach their highest potential, not just the gifted and talented.)

The important thing to recognize if your child is predominantly pitta is to see if those qualities are not being balanced. So ask yourself these questions:

❑ Does my child get in arguments at school?
❑ Does my child have digestive issues, such as acid stomach, diarrhea, or vomiting?
❑ Does my child have severe acne, rash, or other skin inflammations?
❑ Is my child's mood characterized by being irritated and angered at home?
❑ Is my child very uncomfortable in the heat?
❑ Did my daughter start her period early?
❑ Does my child stay up past midnight, reading?
❑ Is my child really competitive in sports, with grades, and with my other children?

If you answer "yes" to these questions about your child's temperament and appearance, it would be a great help to your child's health, life experience, and eventual aging process if you would help her balance pitta through diet and creating a pitta-pacifying environment at home. As usual that means creating an environment for that child that has the opposite qualities of her pitta qualities.

Create a Pitta-Pacifying Home Environment

Creating a pitta-pacifying home environment can be great for everyone, not only the pitta types. A pitta-pacifying home will have the qualities that can cool and calm fiery energy. After a workday or school day, many people—whether predominantly pitta or not—could love and benefit from these tips in the home.

- Learn new things with your child—such as origami, candle making, and knitting—to help satisfy her creativity, without needing to add rewards or competition. Remind her how to enjoy the process and be patient with others.
- Paint the pitta's bedroom soothing, cooling colors, such as the colors you'd find at a spa: light shades of blue and green, like the sky or the ocean. (If she's drawn to very bright and hot colors, use those colors only as sparse accents with a few throw pillows, a fun lamp on her desk, a comfortable reading chair, or a work of art in her favorite colors.)
- When you have to discipline your children, try not to scream. Be aware that if you get heated, your anger will fuel their fire. Stay calm, and yet be real and honest about what you need them to stop doing, to be responsible for, or to understand.
- Spend time outside by moonlight. The moon has a cooling energy. Learn the different constellations together, or read about how explorers knew the map of the sky. Do it with an attitude of relaxation and fun. Learning like this intrigues pitta, and the coolness of the night will help pacify this dosha.

All this is to say, it's so supportive to encourage and celebrate when your child excels, holds leadership roles, and wins in sports. It's also beneficial to create balance when she comes home so that now and later in life she'll be able to balance that pitta fire. She can appreciate its glow and learn how to keep from overheating.

Relax Before Bedtime

It's easy for pittas to keep the momentum going and to want to stay up late. One way to help everyone get to bed before midnight is to stop the stimulating activities early. Movies are stimulating to watch before bedtime, and so is television. If you can make a break between movies or television and going into bed, that could really help pitta transition more smoothly.

Nighttime Activities

Instead of watching movies or playing competitive games at night right before bed, transition from activity to sleep. Consciously make the choice to engage in warm, fun activities together. Read calming bedtime stories together, tell stories about your children's grandparents or about your childhood, encourage your children to journal.

ESSENTIAL

Something you can do as a family is grow plants, vegetables, or herbs. You could use the evening time to talk about the plants, vegetables, and herbs; water them, and observe how they grow and change. Look through recipe books calmly, and think about what you'd like to make with the food you're growing.

When choosing activities to do before bed, try to think of what will not instigate competition or stimulation.

Getting Used to Slowing Down Before Bed

Many single people, as well as families, have a lot of activities each day, and each night might not look the same on the calendar. However, whenever possible, try to stick to the routine of having quiet time before bed. Once everyone, even adults, gets used to carving out time at night to relax before bed, it can become a good habit.

It's really worth it to slow down because pittas can have turbulent dreams, even though they sleep soundly. At the very least, if you cannot make a lot of time to slow down before bed, try this visualization either in a comfortable chair before bed or once you are lying in bed.

NIGHTTIME VISUALIZATION

1. Get comfortable, and close your eyes.
2. Notice yourself sinking into the support of the bed. Take a moment and a few deep breaths to sink into that support.
3. Bring a slight smile to your lips; this will trigger a happy and peaceful feeling.
4. Envision yourself lying down underneath a blue sky.
5. Notice there are just a few clouds, and watch them float slowly across the sky.
6. Envision all the tension melting from your body, sinking down through the bed, down into the earth, melting away. Return your imagination to the blue sky and your breath.
7. After you've done this visualization for several breaths, notice how you feel, and allow yourself to go to sleep.

Visualizations are a wonderful way to calm down after a long day. Another great practice is called yoga nidra, or yogic sleep. For that practice, you'll buy a CD or download yoga nidra onto your iPod. It's a guided relaxation and will help you relax from head to toe, from mind to body.

CHAPTER 10

Keeping Pitta Dosha in Balance

Pitta types love to create, learn, and accomplish. They bring so much innovation and insight into the world. Problem-solving and sharp, the pitta mind is a treasure to behold. Pacifying pitta doesn't mean you have to stop doing interesting things or squelch the bright fire that the world so greatly needs. Balancing this dosha means you'll sustain your energy and learn ways to prevent burning to the point where it's detrimental to your body, mind, or goals that you set for yourself.

Sitting by the Fire

One of the most important first steps to balancing pitta is to get in the habit of observing yourself with as much objectivity as you can. Every day, notice how you're feeling. Check in with yourself throughout the day to see how you're doing. Notice how you react to situations, notice what you're eating, notice what activities you're participating in. Are you doing things to help keep pitta in balance? The first step is to begin to notice how you are feeling and acting. When it comes to pitta's fire, bask in its glow, and also observe it so you can be quick to notice pitta in excess.

Visualization for Understanding Pitta

Imagine that the pitta in you is a like a campfire. You are not the campfire; you are the manager of that fire. Even though pitta is in you, it is not you. You are pure awareness, always, regardless of how the doshas are showing up in you. So, you sit by the fireside of pitta even as it's in your mind and body. As the observer, you don't have to get completely caught up in the fire when pitta's fire is raging with too much heat in you. You can notice the fire is becoming unruly by observing your mental and physical state, and then you'll use your pitta-pacifying skills to bring the fire back into place.

Using the Fire for Transformation

When you sit by the campfire, have you ever noticed that it encourages you to make use of its transformative power? For example, there is a transformation that occurs in food as you cook it. Have you ever been sitting by the campfire in the fire pit of your backyard or enjoying a fire in your fireplace when you become drawn to cook over the open flame? Roasting marshmallows and cooking meals are main activities people are drawn to do when they plan to sit by the fire, even if they could just as easily cook on the nearby stovetop. There's a certain pleasure and excitement connected to cooking over an open flame and witnessing the transformative process. In the same way that you slow down and appreciate the transformative potential in a campfire, step back sometimes and appreciate the transformative power of pitta in you.

Have you also noticed how sitting around a fire can transform your mood? Even if you've had a difficult day or week, when you sit around a campfire, there's a sense of community. People tell stories, share laughter, dance, and relax together around a fire. It transforms coldness and tension into warmth and compassion.

QUOTE

> Ultimately, our potential for cosmic love and dream is made possible by the numinous fire of the universe. Fire energy is perceived by the sense of sight and forms the ability for great vision. This fire is tejas, that which shines and is the moving energy within the billions of atoms in the universe. —Maya Tiwari

Plan to spend some time by the fire, even if it's just by the light of a candle, to remember your inherent potential that is supported by all of the elements and forces of nature. Just as the qualities of fire give energy to your personal unfolding, these same qualities are the powerful solar force that sustains transformation throughout the universe. Stepping back to see the larger picture like this is balancing for a pitta type, who may get so caught up in her momentary achievements that she forgets the larger beautiful picture of life and her participation in it. In fact, pitta types have a very high capacity for understanding broad universal truths; they just have to balance their pitta so they don't limit themselves by focusing only on their personal success and independence.

Foods to Balance Pitta

There are so many options for meals and snacks that will help balance pitta. Some options will appeal to you more than others, so try out different recipes and create your own within the guidelines. The good news is, these foods have been time tested as pitta pacifying, so they are known to support your health. That means, your body will want them and appreciate them, so you will enjoy these foods. There's so much wiggle room for creating the recipes you like best within the choices for a pitta-pacifying effect.

Whole Grains for Pitta

In a pitta diet, it will work for 40 to 50 percent of your diet to be whole grains. Grains can be very satisfying, and there's such a variety of grains that you can choose from, including:

GREAT GRAINS FOR PITTA

- Dry cereal
- Pancakes
- Wheat
- Couscous
- Cooked oats
- White, basmati, and wild rice
- Pasta
- Sprouted grains
- Mochi
- Granola

You can see what a variety you have to choose from. Of course, it's best to choose the nonprocessed foods much more often than processed. Also, find out if you'd do best if you were to avoid gluten. You can find out by simply taking it out of your diet and seeing if your health improves. See if you have more energy, fewer runny noses, fewer headaches, fewer stomachaches, etc. Many people are gluten-intolerant or sensitive without realizing it. When it comes to digesting every grain and food, each person is individual, and you may even change over time. So, the grains listed for pitta are generally grains that sit well with pitta, and yet this doesn't mean all of them will be okay for you. And that's okay. You're experimenting until you find what's best for your body.

Grains that may not work quite so well for pitta are rye, buckwheat, corn bread, quinoa, amaranth, and brown rice. Again, if some of these appeal to you, go ahead and test them out. See if they are okay for you.

Proteins for Pitta

It's really important to have about 10 to 20 percent protein in your diet. The proteins to favor for pitta include lentils (except red lentils), lima beans, aduki beans, black beans, navy beans, soybeans, chickpeas, mung dahl, split peas, tempeh, and cooked tofu. If you are not a vegetarian, white chicken, white turkey, and freshwater fish are good sources of protein for pitta.

FACT

Most health food experts agree that the energy in food gets transferred to your body, so if you eat meat, it's important to know where it came from and how the animal was raised and treated. Others believe that it's not healthy to eat meat at all for many reasons, including the thought that it isn't in keeping with the practice of nonviolence.

While there are so many proteins that support pitta, there are some that aren't as supportive. They include toor dahl, red lentils, and dark meat.

Pitta's Options for Fruits and Veggies

It's best to have 30 to 40 percent of your diet be fruits and vegetables when you're predominantly pitta. See what your body is craving as far as whether to reach for fruit or vegetables. The list is long for fruits and vegetables because they are so good for you. And it's best to choose what's in season. Fruits to favor are apples (not sour apples), apricots, avocadoes, berries (not sour berries), dates, figs, grapes, lemons (see how you do with lemons), limes, kiwi, mangos, melons, oranges, pears, pineapples, plums (sweet), raisins, and watermelons. Vegetables to favor are so numerous; some of them are artichoke, arugula, asparagus, broccoli, brussel sprouts, cabbage, carrots, celery, collards, cucumber, endive, green beans, jicama, kale, lettuce, okra, parsnips, peas, white potatoes, sprouts, winter squash, watercress, and zucchini.

Fruits to reduce in the pitta diet include sour apples, bananas, sour berries, cranberries, grapefruit, peaches, persimmon, and strawberries. Vegetables to reduce are beets, eggplant, horseradish, hot peppers, radishes (raw), raw onion, tomatoes, and turnips.

Nuts, Seeds, and Condiments

Nuts, seeds, and condiments are ways to add texture, flavor, and more prana and nutrient support to your meals. You can sprinkle a handful or two of seeds into soups, on vegetables, in sandwiches, and on pizza. And condiments can be used as dressings, as well as for adding balancing tastes to your meal.

For pitta, soaked and peeled almonds are a great choice. When you want seeds, choose flax, halva, pumpkin, and sunflower. You can also do well with popcorn as long as you go easy on the salt and add some ghee or butter.

Condiments to favor are a little black pepper, dulse, hijiki, kombu, and tamari.

Pittas will feel best by avoiding most nuts, condiments that are salty (such as salt, seaweed, and soy sauce), and condiments that are hot and acidic (such as chili pepper, horseradish, mustard, pickles, and vinegar).

Aromas to Pacify Pitta

Using aromas is a simple way to relax the mind and body. The positive therapeutic effects of aromas are often overlooked in Western culture, even though many people buy scented candles, scented shampoos, and scented deodorant because they are aware that people have responses to scents. If you begin to take advantage of the benefits that your sense of smell can offer you, this will be a whole new area of life that you can draw on to positively support your health.

Balancing Aromas for Pitta

Aromas that balance pitta have the opposite qualities of pitta, so the scents will be sweet, cooling, and calming. Rose, lemongrass, peppermint, gardenia, sandalwood, and jasmine are specific scents to test out and see which you like best.

One of the added benefits to using scents to pacify any dosha, including pitta, is that you can bring your attention to your breath while you inhale and experience the scents. Bringing your awareness to your breath is a very calming practice. If you use a diffuser, after turning it on, lie on your back, and feel the support of the earth. Give yourself at least a five-minute break to just lie down and take a few deep inhales through the nose and long exhales through the mouth. Then, return the breath to normal breathing through the nose only; close your lips, and put on a gentle smile as the scent wafts over you. If you can take this break for more than five minutes, try taking fifteen minutes in this position to cool off and relax. This is something you can do with others, too, because the aroma can fill a room.

FACT

There is a type of Ayurvedic rosewater spray that can be sprayed into the eyes to cool them and reduce redness. This spray is refreshing for all types, especially pitta, because it's cooling, and the scent of rose is sweet. Rose also acts as an anti-inflammatory to help reduce puffiness. Keep a bottle at home and another at the office to use after staring at the computer screen too long.

Aromas Before Bedtime

Pitta dreams can be violent. By balancing pitta throughout the day, you can help alleviate the frequency of difficult dreams. Using aromatherapy earlier in the day and also before bedtime can help calm the mind. Lavender is a scent that is often used in bedrooms, bathrooms, and spas to soothe anxiety and an overactive mind. Try using a lavender spray in your room, lavender in your diffuser, or a lavender-scented candle as part of your bedtime routine (blow out the candle before falling asleep).

Activities to Pacify Pitta

Everything you do affects your health: your thoughts, meals, and activities all affect your mood, your physical health, and how gracefully you age. Allow yourself to be very intentional about what you do. You can still be spontaneous at times, and do things that may throw you a little off-kilter. That's part of life, and you don't have to be completely rigid. That being said, if you can follow guidelines for your type more often than not, that's a very good start. And the more smart choices you decide to make, the more you will notice that your mood, your productivity, and your physical health improve.

Choose When to Be Vigorous

Pittas can be drawn to vigorous and heat-producing activity because it helps them burn off steam, which is a good thing for pittas to do. Early morning is an ideal time for pitta types to go for a run, play tennis, or ride a bike.

If you are pitta, it's best to gravitate toward vigorous activities when it feels like you're burning off some steam to release the heat rather than doing vigorous activity to heat you up more when you already feel your pitta is high. It might take some time for you to learn the difference. Practice checking in with yourself after your workout or vigorous activity: Do you feel more balanced, or do you feel hotheaded, angry, and overstimulated? If it's the latter, you could be burning yourself out. You'll also be able to tell based on the physical symptoms of unbalanced pitta that will show up in your body, your mind, and your relationships if you are overdoing it.

QUESTION

Are there ways to keep pitta balanced and do vigorous activity?
Choose not to do vigorous activities during pitta time of day, or if you must, limit those activities to about an hour. Stay hydrated (add coconut water to your list of refreshing drinks), and take time to cool off afterward with gentle yoga postures, meditation, a cooling shower, a swim, or pitta-pacifying pranayama.

Vigorous activity is absolutely fine for pitta if you also do things to create balance. Choose your favorite ways to cool off, eat well for your type, and practice habits that are peaceful and compassionate for your mind. If you make sure to balance your fire, you can still participate in vigorous activities and debates and stay healthy.

Walk a Labyrinth

Labyrinths are not mazes. A labyrinth is a pattern made of one winding path that begins at the starting point (the mouth), turns back and forth, and ends up in the center. It is unicursal, which means it's just one path in and the same path out. When you walk the labyrinth, you start at the mouth, follow the path in, and pause in the center. Then, you follow the same path out. As you walk it, you have no choices to make about which way to go. It leads you, and there are no dead ends. You will always make it to the center if you keep following the path.

Labyrinths have been around for millennia. You can find them in churches and in a variety of beautiful outdoor settings. You can even find small versions inscribed on the ruins of ancient places of worship: people would finger-walk the labyrinth before entering the building to pray. Walking the pattern of the labyrinth is known to help you feel centered.

SUGGESTIONS FOR WALKING THE LABYRINTH

1. Step up to the mouth. Set an intention for your walk. If you're feeling your pitta is aggravated, resolve to find peace and calm during your walk.
2. Enter the labyrinth. Walk slowly. Follow your breath with each step. Inhale on one step, exhale on the next.
3. Allow this rhythmic breathing and walking to calm and soothe you.
4. See if you can slow down your breathing and your pace.
5. Once you get to the center, pause. Take deep breaths. If the labyrinth is outdoors, really notice your surroundings.
6. Close your eyes. With your eyes closed, watch the breath flow in and out.
7. Remember your intention to feel peace and calm.
8. Slowly walk back the way you came in, with your attention on your steps and your surroundings.
9. After you exit the labyrinth, turn and take a moment to appreciate what's transpired for you.
10. Take a moment after walking the labyrinth to rest. Notice any changes that have occurred in how you're feeling.

Walking a labyrinth can be done in so many ways. Instead of setting an intention to find peace and calm, you can set any intention you would like. You can also walk it without an intention and just see what happens. Because of the way the labyrinth winds back and forth, it has the physiological effect of balancing the energy between the two hemispheres of the brain. This produces a calming effect. This calming effect is a wonderful balance for pitta.

Yoga for Balancing Pitta

The following yoga and pranayama sequences are designed for pitta types by Janna Delgado, a yoga and Ayurvedic specialist at Kripalu Center for Yoga & Health. Yoga is not "one size fits all," Janna explains, meaning that you can choose particular postures and practices depending on what you need for balance. For example, a vata practice should be steady and grounding to keep you stable; a pitta practice should have an internal focus on surrender and nonjudgment to cool your competitive nature; and a kapha practice should be active and warming to awaken your energy.

Because pitta types have a tendency to overheat by pushing themselves way too hard, they benefit most from a cooling, calming, and relaxed yoga practice. Softer poses help reduce the heat and emotional intensity that pitta types are prone to. To pacify a pitta imbalance, the key is to remember that less is more. Practice surrendering rather than striving, and focus on acceptance rather than judgment.

Warm Up

Always begin your yoga practice with a warm-up. Keep it moderate— nothing too heating or challenging. For example, a great warm-up for pitta types would be to rotate and loosen up all of the joints in the body. Be sure to include your ankles, knees, hips, wrists, elbows, shoulders, neck, and spine.

Once warmed up, become still, soften your gaze on the horizon, and bring your awareness to your breath. Take a few minutes to cultivate a steady and slow breathing rhythm. Once you have established your breath, begin to slow down and lengthen your exhalations by drawing your navel toward the spine as you breathe out. This technique of elongated, slow-motion exhalations should be used throughout the following sequence to help calm your body and nervous system.

Standing Wide Angle Forward Fold

Before doing any postures, it's important to know the benefits and the contraindications. Benefits of Standing Wide Angle Forward Fold include the following: the pose cools and circulates abdominal energy, it calms an overheated brain, and it sends excess heat down the energy channels in the legs and into the earth. Contraindication for wide angle forward fold is that those suffering from lower-back issues should either avoid this pose or keep the knees bent while practicing it.

HOW TO PRACTICE WIDE ANGLE FORWARD FOLD

1. Stand with your feet 3 to 4 feet apart with hands on your hips.
2. Bring your feet parallel to each other and press the outer edges of your feet firmly into the floor.
3. Firm up your thigh muscles.
4. Inhale and lift your chest.
5. Hinging at the hips, exhale and lift your tailbone as you fold forward, keeping your spine long.
6. When your torso is parallel to the floor, place your hands on the floor directly below your shoulders. (Place your hands on blocks or thick books as a modification. Or, if the backs of your legs or spine are tight, bend your knees.)
7. Distribute your weight evenly between your hands and feet. Work to lengthen your arms and legs.
8. Widen your shoulder blades across your back and draw your shoulders away from your ears.
9. Gaze straight down and lengthen your spine from the tip of your tailbone through the crown of your head.
10. Stay in the pose for five to ten deep breaths, with an emphasis on longer exhalations for a cooling effect.

You can proceed directly to the next posture, Twisting Wide Angle Forward Fold, or come out and rest first. To come out of the pose, press your feet into the floor and bring your hands to your hips. Inhale and press your tailbone down toward the floor, as you lift your torso up to vertical. Step your feet together, close your eyes, and feel the effects of the pose.

Twisting Wide Angle Forward Fold

One benefit of twisting is that it massages the organs of digestion, which are where pitta lives in the body. Twists also help you avoid overheating or becoming overly aggressive because they wring out excess heat. The contraindications are for those suffering from issues of the spine and pregnant women: these people should avoid this pose.

TWISTING WIDE ANGLE FORWARD FOLD

1. Come into Standing Wide Angle Forward Fold, as described above, with your hands on the floor (or blocks) below your shoulders, your feet firmly planted on the floor, and your torso elongated.
2. Lift your left hand and place it on the floor on the outside of your right hand, pressing your palm firmly down into the floor. If there is tension in your lower back or legs, bend your knees a bit.
3. Exhale and sweep your right hand up toward the ceiling. Revolve your spine and extend up through your arm.
4. Breathe deeply for five to ten breaths, elongating your exhalations to help decompress pitta.
5. Release by lowering your right arm on an inhalation.
6. Return to Standing Wide Angle Pose for one complete breath.
7. Repeat the above steps, twisting to the other side (your left side) for five to ten breaths, focusing on long exhalations to calm your nervous system.
8. To come out, release your left arm toward the floor and return to Standing Wide Angle Forward Fold.
9. Place your hands on your hips, inhale, and press your tailbone down toward the floor as you lift the torso up to vertical.
10. Step your feet together. Pause to feel the effects of the forward fold and twist.

Fish

This is a heart-opening pose. The benefit is that it helps pitta types to soften and cultivate compassion toward themselves and others. When you are overheated or irritable, this pose opens up the abdomen and solar plexus, allowing for the movement of energy to cool excess pitta.

Contraindications are for those with uncontrolled high or low blood pressure, migraines, or insomnia, and those who suffer from low back or neck injury: these people should not practice this posture.

FISH POSTURE

1. Lie on your back on the floor.
2. Slide your hands underneath your buttocks, palms facing down.
3. Keep your legs straight and active. Flex your feet so your toes point toward the ceiling.
4. Draw your elbows in close toward your rib cage and press your elbows and forearms firmly into the floor.
5. Inhale and lift your upper back and shoulders away from the floor, while maintaining contact between the back of your head and the floor. If you feel any discomfort, come out of the pose. Otherwise, work to keep the elbows and forearms firmly pressed down into the floor.
6. Keep your throat soft and your breath steady. On your exhale, draw your navel back to the spine to help elongate your exhalations.
7. Take five to ten deep breaths.
8. To come out of the pose, exhale and release your torso and shoulders back down to the floor.
9. Carefully draw your knees into your chest and relax for a few breaths.

Reclined Twist

This twist is great for pitta types because it's calming and not overly heating. Remember, too, that twists release excess pitta from the digestive organs, which are the seat of pitta in the body. This pose is contraindicated if you are pregnant or experiencing any hip or back pain. In that case, stop practicing twists and consult a physician.

RECLINED TWIST

1. To begin, lie on your back with your knees bent and your feet on the floor. If there is tension in your neck and shoulders, place a folded blanket or thin pillow under your head.
2. Take a few moments to breathe deeply to melt away any tension. Let go. Feel the muscles in the back of your body soften and spread out as they sink down onto the floor.
3. Draw both knees into your chest.
4. Take your arms out to the sides, on the floor, perpendicular to your body, with palms facing up. Inhale deeply.
5. Exhale slowly as you release your hips and let your knees drop over to the right side.
6. Place your right hand on your left knee, keeping both shoulders flat on the floor.
7. Turn your head to the left. If this is not comfortable, then keep your head centered.
8. Soften and surrender as you breathe quietly here. Without straining, draw your navel toward your spine on each exhalation to create a slow-motion and complete exhalation.
9. Take five to ten breaths, drawing your awareness inward to focus on the sensation of your breath.
10. Return to center on an inhalation and repeat on the other side.

When you've completed both sides, draw both knees to your chest and rock gently from side to side for a few breaths. Then release your arms and legs on the floor, and relax for a few breaths to receive the full benefit of the twists.

Reclined Bound Angle Variation

This calming, cooling, and restorative pose eases general fatigue, releases excess heat from the inner thighs and groin, boosts immunity, and invites pitta types to drop into a quieter and more introspective space. This pose is not for those who have a serious eye condition, such as glaucoma, or for those sufferers of neck, back, knee, or groin conditions.

RECLINED BOUND ANGLE VARIATION

1. Start seated with your left hip against a wall, then recline back onto your forearms.
2. With one smooth movement, swing both legs up onto the wall and release your torso and head gently down onto the floor.
3. Scoot your buttocks toward the wall until they rest a few inches away from it.
4. Bend your knees, touch the soles of the feet together, and let the outer edges of your feet slide down the wall until your heels rest comfortably above your groin.
5. Take your arms out to your sides, on the floor, palms up.
6. Let your shoulder blades melt away from the spine and sink down to the floor.
7. Relax and soften your whole body.
8. Breathe comfortably with extended exhalations to help you relax.
9. Use your breath to create spaciousness and ease in your body and mind.
10. Stay in the pose for five to fifteen minutes.
11. To come out of the pose, draw your knees together, roll onto your side, and come into a fetal position.
12. Take a few breaths to absorb the aftereffects of the pose.

Cooldown

Pitta types need plenty of time for relaxation and integration at the end of a practice to allow accumulated pitta to completely release. Be sure to rest in savasana, lying on your back, for at least fifteen minutes with a soft, relaxed breath. Allow yourself to completely let go and surrender into stillness.

Pranayama for Pitta Pacification

Pranayama refers to breathing exercises. When you practice pranayama, it helps if you are in a quiet, clean, and tranquil location with good ventilation.

Practice the following pranayama on an empty stomach, in a comfortable seated position, either on the floor or in a chair, with the spine, neck, and head erect. Clothing should be loose and comfortable.

ESSENTIAL

Avoid strain with all pranayama practices. Do not practice pranayama during times of illness. If you experience negative side effects, physical or emotional, discontinue the practice and consult with a qualified yoga teacher or a physician.

Three-Part Breath (Dirgha)

Three-part breath is good for all doshas, and when done with a focus on long, relaxed exhalations it is especially good for calming the mind and nervous system. Avoid this exercise if you have had recent surgery or injury in your torso or head.

THREE-PART BREATH (DIRGHA)

1. Sit comfortably with a long spine.
2. Seal your lips and relax your forehead, jaw, and belly.
3. Begin to take steady, long breaths in and out through your nostrils.
4. Let your breath slow down so much that you can feel your belly, rib cage, then chest expand and contract with each inhalation and exhalation.
5. Take a few minutes to establish a relaxed and even breathing rhythm.
6. Next, begin to slow down and extend your exhalations, allowing them to become longer than your inhalations. To help lengthen your exhalations, gently contract your abdominal muscles as you breathe out.
7. Without straining, draw your navel back to the spine to create slow-motion exhalations.
8. Gradually build your exhalations to last twice as long as your inhalations. Stay relaxed as you gently contract your abdominal muscles to squeeze the air out of your lungs. Breathing this way helps to release strong emotions, such as anger, frustration, and impatience.
9. Continue for three to five minutes.

Lunar Breath/Left Nostril Breath (Chandra Bheda)

Lunar breath helps to expel excess pitta. By directing the breath through the left nostril, which is associated with the cooling energy of the moon, the mind and body become soothed and relaxed. If you suffer from low blood pressure, depression, colds, flu, or any other respiratory conditions, avoid this pranayama.

LUNAR BREATH/LEFT NOSTRIL BREATH

1. Sit comfortably with a long spine.
2. Hold up your right hand and fold your index and middle fingers into the palm of your hand, keeping the thumb, ring finger, and pinky extended.
3. Seal your right nostril with your thumb and take a slow and complete breath in through your left nostril.
4. Seal your left nostril with your ring finger, release your thumb, and exhale out of the right nostril.
5. Repeat this sequence—inhaling through your left nostril and exhaling through your right.
6. Continue for three to five minutes.

In addition to calming your mind and cooling your entire body, this breathing exercise relaxes your muscles, promotes tranquility, and increases introspection.

Cooling Breath (Shitali)

Cooling Breath is done by inhaling through your mouth and exhaling through your nose. This breathing practice should be done gently and without force. It is best to practice either early or late in the day, when the air is cool, to keep pitta from overheating. Avoid this exercise if you are experiencing extreme cold or hypothermia.

COOLING BREATH (SHITALI)

1. Sit comfortably with a long spine.
2. Purse your lips, stick your tongue out, and curl it lengthwise, into the shape of a straw.
3. Inhale slowly through the straw and fill your lungs completely.
4. Relax your tongue and draw it back into your mouth, seal your lips, and exhale through your nose very slowly.
5. Repeat this cycle, inhaling though your curled tongue, closing your mouth, and exhaling through your nostrils, for three to five minutes.

If you can't curl your tongue, just keep it relaxed in your mouth and inhale through pursed lips.

Integration

When finished with your pranayama practice, return to normal breathing for a minute or two, then lie down in savasana, on your back with eyes closed, for several minutes to allow for integration. Pranayama is a natural, effective way to help cool down and keep pitta in balance.

CHAPTER 11

Understanding Kapha

Kapha types are known for their sweet, forgiving, and stable nature. If you are predominantly kapha, you tend to do things slowly. Your general approach to activity can be best described as slow and steady, and you're known for physical endurance. Staying active is one of the best things you can do to keep your kapha in balance. Mentally, once you learn something, you remember it. So, don't be discouraged if it takes you a little longer to learn something than it takes your vata or pitta friends.

What Is Kapha?

Kapha is of the elements earth and water. Kapha's qualities are stable, oily, heavy, dense, smooth, and cool. A kapha type will remind you of Mother Earth: she emanates a nurturing, tolerant energy, with a calming sense of stability.

Recognizing the Kapha Body Type

Kapha types tend to have nice curves and some excess body weight. Their bodies are heavy and strong. Kapha's skin appears soft, smooth, oily, clear, and pale. Their eyes are sensual, black or blue, clear, big, and bright. Hair is blond or jet-black, wavy, shiny, and abundant.

When trying to determine if you or a loved one has the characteristics of a kapha body, see if any of these descriptions apply.

KAPHA BODY TYPE CHECKLIST

❑ I have thick muscles, strong bones, and a large body frame.
❑ I gain weight easily, and it's very hard to take it off.
❑ I have long, thick eyelashes.
❑ My skin is often cold and clammy.
❑ My eyes are large and round.
❑ I am prone to getting congested in my head, throat, and chest.

If you say "That's me!" when you read most of these attributes, you are noticing kapha qualities. This isn't enough to determine, yet, if kapha is the only dosha dominant in your constitution. You may have a significant amount of the attributes of another dosha, too. Everyone has some of all three doshas at work in the body. So, a more comprehensive Ayurvedic questionnaire and a meeting with an Ayurvedic specialist will help you determine how predominant kapha is in your personal constitution.

Kapha Mind

Kaphas are slow to learn, but once they learn something they will remember it. They are peaceful by nature and very forgiving. Kaphas develop attachments to people and things, which is why they tend to store and save items more than other people will. They can be prone to envy and greed if kapha is out of balance.

Ojas, Kapha's Subtle Energy

Just as vata and pitta have their subtle energies (prana and tejas, respectively), kapha has a subtle energy: ojas. Ojas is the essence that remains after your digestion and assimilation of food, thoughts, and impressions. If you are able to digest well, then ojas will be sustained in you. It will keep the vital organs and tissues of your body healthy. Ojas provides endurance for both the body and the mind.

It is said that among its many sustaining attributes, ojas lubricates the nerves of the nervous system, so nervous breakdowns, for example, signal low ojas. Ojas is needed for emotional tranquility.

How to Recognize Kapha Imbalance

There are physical and emotional signs of kapha imbalance. It's important to balance kapha and catch these signs early because too much kapha engenders a kind of lethargy that can be hard to move through, making it harder to get back in balance. Fortunately, as with all doshas, you know what to do: start doing activities, thinking thoughts, and eating foods that have the opposite qualities that kapha has.

Kapha's Physical Symptoms of Imbalance

When kapha is in excess, you will feel lethargic. You will need naps, you will have a difficult time getting out of bed in the morning, and you will gain weight. You may start to have mucous drainage, coughs, and sinus headaches. A general sense of inertia and inability to motivate yourself to physically move will increase as the kapha tips more and more off balance.

See if these apply to you:

PHYSICAL SIGNS OF YOUR KAPHA IN EXCESS

- You drink at least two cups of coffee during the day, and there is no effect.

- You go to sleep early, you sleep in, and still you're feeling low energy all day.
- You're craving sweets, eating sweets, and gaining weight.
- Your body is discharging mucus.

These could be signs of a kapha imbalance. If you notice these signs, start changing your food choices and activities to balance kapha. The fastest and simplest thing you can do is to modify what you eat: that has an immediate impact on the body.

Gluten intolerance can produce very similar effects to kapha being out of balance, or even other doshas being out of balance. So it's very important to find out what you are allergic to, either by consulting your doctors or by taking things out of your diet and seeing if your symptoms improve. For many people, it's best to avoid gluten.

Sometimes you will just be tired and lethargic because you've been burning yourself out. If you aren't sure, give yourself a few days of rest, being sure to hydrate well. If the symptoms persist, this could include both a kapha imbalance and also other issues that need to be addressed. So talk to your doctors and healers if you're noticing lethargy and weight gain.

Kapha's Mental and Emotional Signs of Imbalance

Kapha is by nature loving, caring, grounding, and forgiving, and when kapha is in excess it can turn into jealousy and feelings of needing to cling onto something and someone. If you're starting to feel jealous and clingy, this could be your sign that your kapha is out of balance.

Effects of Long-Term Kapha Imbalance

Every doshic imbalance has particular long-term effects. When kapha is out of balance, it creates the logical kinds of difficulties on the body that you would imagine from its qualities of stable, oily, heavy, dense, smooth, and cool.

Obesity

If you sit often because of work, munch throughout the day on food, watch a lot of TV when you're not working, and sleep a lot, you could very likely be increasing your kapha. You will notice the effects in weight gain and apathy, which may make you feel unmotivated to change these habits. Constant sitting and eating can result in obesity, which is very difficult on the organs, bones, and entire body.

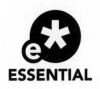

ESSENTIAL

For anybody, sitting for long periods of time isn't healthy. For kapha types especially, it's good to get in some movement every day. After work is a great time to go for a nice, brisk walk—you'll get exercise and walk off frustration. If you can't walk outdoors, walk around the mall. Don't interrupt the walk with shopping, though. Shop afterward.

Catching weight gain early and seeing a doctor about it before becoming obese is ideal. If you are already very overweight, or obese, talk to an Ayurvedic specialist and a doctor, and they can help you shed the pounds. You will have to work at it, as everyone does, but you can do it! It is very possible, especially with the support of those who know about health and nutrition.

Other Conditions That May Be Signs of Excess Kapha

These conditions may also be the result of excess kapha in you:

- High cholesterol
- Cataracts
- Diabetes

If you have any of these conditions, your Ayurvedic specialist will want to know how long you've had them, what you are doing about them, and if there is a history of these conditions in your family. She and your doctor will help you, taking all things about you and your history into consideration. If you don't show signs of these but you have a lot of kapha in your constitution and a family history, these are conditions you may want to be aware of so you can be proactive by keeping your kapha in check. Keeping your doshas balanced by eating well, getting exercise, and having fun in your life is a great start.

Kapha Time of Day, Year, and Life

Whether or not you have a predominance of kapha in your constitution, you have some kapha in you. And the natural world outside is characterized by the qualities of kapha at certain times of day and year. If you don't have a lot of kapha in you, you can use these times of day, year, and life to help create balance in you. Learn to sink into the qualities of these times of day—allowing them to affect you.

Kapha Time of Day

In the morning, kapha time is from 6–10 A.M. Some of the benefits of kapha are that it helps build up the body and lubricate the joints, which is ideal for this time of day as you wake up and get ready for your day. The morning kapha hours are the perfect time to engage in exercise. Your warm-ups are meant for lubricating the joints, and your morning walk or exercise will help get your muscles awake and ready to support you throughout your day. These goals are supported by kapha's lubricating and body-building qualities.

ESSENTIAL

If you are experiencing a kapha disorder or if you are predominantly kapha, the morning kapha time is the best time to do self-massage. A deep massage is best for your type, and you can use corn oil or no oil at all. Remember, kapha is already oily by nature.

From 6–10 P.M. are the kapha hours of the evening. These hours are great hours for you to start winding down and preparing for sleep. You can tap in to kapha's stable, sweet, and heavy qualities to help you transition from the action of the day into a mind–body state that's conducive to sweet dreams.

Kapha Time of Year

Kapha time of year is the springtime, when the cold and dryness of winter begins to melt into liquid. The rain pours, adding moisture and creating heavy mud. Mother Nature comes into bloom, and the sweet sounds of the birds singing heralds the kapha morning time.

Because this is the kapha time of year, people are prone to getting colds, sinus infections, and even the flu. To help stay healthy, do a spring cleanse for yourself. Help expel what's been built up inside of you from the winter months. For a spring cleanse, talk to your Ayurvedic practitioner for supervision. If you cannot do a thorough cleanse, here are a few suggestions to help support the release of built-up toxins in your body, as you transition from winter to spring.

GENTLE ONE-WEEK SPRING CLEANSE

1. Do the morning routine each day that purifies the senses. (It's best to keep this up yearlong for all the doshas.)
2. Take a brisk morning walk, and breathe in the fresh air of the new season.
3. Eat lightly and very cleanly for a week: eat whole foods for your type; sip warm water throughout the day to flush your system; avoid snacking, drinking alcohol or coffee, and eating candy.
4. Drink a cup of cumin, coriander, and ginger tea either in the morning or in the evening during kapha time. (Put ¼ teaspoon cumin, ¼ teaspoon coriander, and ¼ teaspoon ginger in a teapot, pour boiling water into the pot, and let it steep five minutes. Strain, and drink.)
5. Take triphala before bedtime, at least one hour after eating. (Put ½ teaspoon in a teapot, add boiling water, and steep for ten minutes. Strain and drink.) Triphala is a very mild and effective laxative. It's all-natural, and nonhabit forming.
6. Journal before going to bed, releasing any stuck emotions or thoughts that have built up for you.
7. Go to bed at an appropriate time. If you don't feel tired, give yourself a soothing oil massage before getting into bed. Then, go to bed and relax. You may be more tired than you realize until you get into bed. Vatas, go to bed by 10 P.M.; pittas, go to bed by 11 P.M.; kaphas, go to bed by midnight.
8. Each morning when you awake, let the first thing you drink be a tall glass of warm water to help with elimination.

Before or after doing your own personal cleanse, clean the entire home. Get rid of clothes you haven't worn in a year or two, and do a deep cleaning of the entire house. Put the heavy winter clothes to the back of the closet, and bring out the lighter, brighter springtime clothes.

Kapha Time of Life

The kapha years are your earliest years. Babies and children are in their kapha time. It's the time of life when healthy babies will be chubby, they will be attached to their mother, and they will be growing (which kapha supports). You will notice that children produce a lot of mucus, too, which is part of kapha's support of the growth process.

QUOTE

For kids, this lubrication is extremely significant because it supports their elastic growth—up to a foot each year. The amount of lubrication in a kid's body is one reason why a seven-year-old child can slide down a set of stairs laughing with each bump whereas an eighty-year-old would simply break. —Dr. John Douillard

As children are growing it's important to notice how their kapha is affecting them. For example, if the mucous production gets too high and they are developing chronic colds, you will want to help balance out their kapha with the kapha balancing tips for meals and activities.

If you notice your child is gaining weight, sleeps a lot, and has a high capacity for compassion, all of these are kapha qualities and consistent with this time of life. Because of this, your child will need your acceptance that these are the natural tendencies in this time of life, and you can help him stay in balance by helping provide the opposite qualities in food and lifestyle. This is a perfect time of life to teach him healthy eating and exercise habits—and exercise can mean playing sports, playing fun active games outside, and taking nice walks together.

Kapha in Balance

Kapha in balance gives the world cohesion, compassion, nurturance, stability, moisture, calm, and sensuality.

Kapha's Glow

Kapha in balance shows up as kindness, calm, and compassion. With big eyes, thick lashes, and a rounded figure, the kapha type appears soft, sensual, and at peace. Her skin has a glow: radiant, smooth, and plump like a child's. And her hair, thick and oily, shimmers in the sunlight.

In balance, a kapha's personality is sincerely friendly, generous with support, and forgiving. Her smile brightens up the room. Her eyes have an unassuming gleam like the afternoon sparkle on the lake (if blue-eyed) or the sheen of the midnight sky (if black).

Kapha as Mother Nature

Kapha types in balance are known to be Mother Nature incarnate. When you have a kapha beloved in your life, you may feel as though he is holding you, seeing you, looking out for you, and making sure you are doing okay.

QUOTE

> Kapha's basic energy sustains everything. She is the principle foundation upon which all the blocks of existence are built. Kapha is the archetypal Mother Earth. The kapha person is the classic synthesis of stoical grace, calm, and sensuality. —Maya Tiwari

As the archetypal Mother Earth, kaphas have the grounded and unctuous energy that provide balance to the mobility, and speed that can get out of hand in pitta and vata. Because everyone has each of the doshas inside, if you're not feeling connected to your kapha, here are a few ways to help you connect to your naturally grounded and calm center.

MAKE SPICED ALMOND MILK

1. Pour ½ cup almond milk and ½ cup spring water into a pot on the stove.
2. Add a pinch of nutmeg.
3. Add a pinch of unrefined brown sugar.
4. Heat until warm, stirring occasionally.
5. Pour into a mug, and slowly enjoy.

To really enjoy this spiced milk, take time to do nothing else while you sip it. Don't watch TV, talk on the phone, or check e-mail. Sit back on your couch or favorite chair, and savor the warmth of the liquid as it passes through your mouth and into your body. Take in its sweet, soothing qualities. Get acquainted with the kapha in you.

Another activity that can help you connect to the earth and water elements in nature is to take a walk and to be conscious of bringing your senses to the experience. In other words, don't think of all the to-dos and worries while you're on the walk. Allow your mind to relax and drop into the sensory experiences of the outdoors.

LOOK FOR ANIMALS

1. Go to a park, where you're bound to find trees, bushes, and rocks.
2. Take a walk through the park with others, and walk slowly enough that you can be on the lookout for animals.
3. Listen for sounds, stand still, and see what you can find inside trees and bushes.
4. Bring your eyes to the ground, looking for the animals who scurry on land.
5. If you don't see or hear any animals on your walk, listen for other sounds. Listen for wind in the trees, running water, or rustling in the bushes. Allow your senses to help you connect to nature.
6. Now take in the scents. Notice what you can smell in trees, flowers, and the air: notice where there is fragrance. Kapha is located in the sense of smell and the sense of taste, so if it's the appropriate time of year, combine this walk with berry picking. Then you can also taste the wonders of nature.

Use your imagination for ways to connect to nature, and allow your family or friends to come along with you. Especially if you need to connect to your kapha qualities, choose to bring along a calming, peaceful, and supportive person in your life.

Ask Friends to Join You

Because of your many attractive kapha qualities, including your tolerant, forgiving, and kind nature, others will enjoy being friends with you and will learn from your sweet ways. So don't be shy about asking friends and family to join you for a regular walking date.

Morning Walks

People of all constitutions benefit from a brisk morning walk. It's a wonderful way to connect to nature first thing in the morning. The benefit of making a walking date with a friend is that it will help you stick to it, since kapha's tendency is to stay put if given the choice.

QUOTE

> Take the power to choose what you want to do and do it well. Take the power to love what you want in life and love it honestly. Take the power to walk in the forest and be a part of nature. Take the power to control your own life. No one else can do it for you. Take the power to make your life happy. —Susan Polis Schutz

One of the best things that a kapha can practice is taking the steps to do what he wants to do in his life. And he can begin to rev up that momentum by taking those first steps in the morning, outside, with a friend or family member.

Make It a Mexican Night

Kaphas like to eat, so why not organize a meal with friends that helps keep you in balance? Organize a potluck, asking if people could follow a Mexican-food theme for the night. Or go out to a Mexican restaurant, and be sure that you order some hot food to balance kapha. Here are some ingredients to favor on Mexican night out:

- Hot peppers, chili peppers, bell peppers
- Onions
- Corn
- Garlic
- Black beans, lima beans, navy beans, pinto beans

Good Mexican restaurants will absolutely have what you need for some heat and to warm up that internal fire. If you host a potluck, here's a refried beans recipe you can make on your own.

Refried Beans

1. Rinse 2 cups of uncooked pinto beans, and pick out any debris.

2. Put the pinto beans in a pot. Pour water over the beans until the water is an inch higher than the tops of the beans.

3. Bring the beans to a boil, then drain the water. Keep the beans in the pot.

4. Cover the beans with about 2 inches of water, bring to a boil, and simmer until the beans are soft. (This can take from 2 to 4 hours.) Add boiling water as necessary to keep the beans boiling.

5. After the beans are soft, sauté 2 tablespoons of minced garlic in corn oil. Do this for 1 to 2 minutes in a skillet big enough to hold the beans, too.

6. Once the garlic is sautéed, add the softened beans and 1 to 2 tablespoons of the liquid they were simmering in.

7. Mash the beans, adding more liquid as necessary for the consistency you'd like.

8. Continue to cook and stir the mixture until it's very warm and a creamy consistency: about 2 to 5 more minutes.

9. Garnish with pepper and cilantro.

Beans, garlic, and pepper are wonderful for the kapha constitution, and using corn oil is the best oil for kaphas. Cilantro is a perfect garnish for all constitutions. It's an herb with many healing benefits, and it helps digestion—what a great support for kapha! (For other doshas, you can use other oils instead of corn oil for sautéing garlic—try olive oil or ghee.)

CHAPTER 12

How to Balance Kapha

...ha, you naturally avoid rushing ...ne thing to the next. So take ...ortant role in the world that ...l, and calming presence. Also, ...and happiness, you'll need to ...by adding movement to your ...ere are plenty of ways to keep ...n find ways to enjoy doing it!

Getting Unstuck

If your kapha starts to go out of balance toward excess, you may start slipping slowly into a lethargic state without realizing it until you're in it. Then you'll be feeling sluggish and unmotivated. When you realize this is happening, the good news is that you can take actions to help remedy the heavy feelings. You don't have to stay stuck in the mud.

Believe This Can Change

If you notice that you're feeling as though you're moving through glue or molasses in your life, you can take steps to change that feeling. What you eat, what you do, and what you think have a direct impact on how you are feeling physically and emotionally. You can change how you're feeling within moments through yoga, meditation, your next meal, or a good pep talk from someone who cares about you. When you believe that you can bring change to your attitude and physical health by what you eat, think, and do, you tap in to an important aspect of true healing.

FACT

Motivational words have a significant impact on your mood and physical health. Have you ever noticed how reading an inspiring quotation or getting a card in the mail can change your state of mind? The mind switches from moment to moment, and you can turn your focus to inspirational and supportive thoughts, which in turn help the body de-stress and thrive.

If you're feeling very sluggish and unmotivated, first know that change is possible. Let your Ayurvedic specialist know how you're feeling, and he can help. In the meantime, just take one step at a time. Find ways to deal with the emotions (through therapy, support, journaling, etc.). And, for the next meal you make, be sure it's balancing for your dosha. Avoid the foods you know will weigh you down. And call a friend to see if you can have a date soon— go for a walk together, get moving!

Do Something Special to Switch Your Mood

If you're feeling heavy and unmotivated, see if you can take a five-minute break to do something special for yourself to switch your mood. Here are some ideas.

FIVE-MINUTE MOOD CHANGERS

- Make a cup of tea. There are so many varieties of tea, and many companies are making their teas in transparent tea bags with wonderfully fresh and innovative blends inside. Once you find out what teas you like, keep some in your office and home. And when you need a pick-me-up, take a tea break to shift your mood.
- Stop what you're doing (or not doing), and write down something that you'd rather be doing instead, whether it's being with your children, going to a movie, or going to the beach. Make it simple, and also something you'd really like to do. Then write down the steps you have to take to make it happen. Resolve to find time to do each step, as you can.
- Stand up and shake it off. Stand up where you are and feel your feet firmly on the ground. Then lift one foot at a time and shake your leg while you inhale and exhale three times. (If balancing is hard for you, hold on to the back of a chair so you don't fall.) After you shake out both legs, shake out your arms for three long breaths.

Sometimes the best thing you can do is make a momentary shift in what you're doing, and that can change your mood. Of course, if your kapha is in excess, it will take more effort to really change your psychological and physical states in a sustained way. So just take one step at a time; "one moment at a time" is the tried-and-true method: one meal, one brisk walk, and one new adventure at a time.

Foods to Balance Kapha

Because kaphas often need to build up their digestive fire, it's important to become aware of what you can eat for support. There are many, many options for you to choose from. There are also some foods to avoid; that way what you eat won't undermine your other efforts toward feeling well.

Grains for Kapha

There are a great many grains for kapha to choose from, including barley, buckwheat, corn, couscous, dry cereal, granola, millet, muesli, oat bran, dry oats, rye, and sprouted wheat bread. It's best for kapha to go easy on amaranth, quinoa, and basmati rice. Avoid rice flour, whole wheat flour (breads and pasta), brown rice, rice cakes, and wheat. The rule of thumb is, if it's sweet it will increase kapha. (If you like to eat pasta, occasionally soba or udon noodles are best choices for you.)

ESSENTIAL

You'll want to avoid foods with the same qualities as kapha, such as heavy, cool, and oily. So when in doubt, think about the qualities of the foods. For example, cold cereals are fine because they are dry and therefore can balance the moist kapha quality. Avoid cucumbers which are cooling and moist.

Kapha and Protein-Rich Foods

Beans are wonderful for kapha. Beans for you are aduki, black, chickpeas (black or yellow), red lentils, lima beans, navy beans, and pinto beans. It's best to limit black-eyed peas, mung dahl, and tofu. Soybeans and miso are not supportive for kapha types.

If you are going to eat meat, according to Dr. Lad, white chicken, eggs, freshwater fish, shrimp, white turkey, and venison are recommended.

Kapha and Vegetables

Many vegetables support kapha. Buy locally grown and organic as often as possible. Great choices for kapha include arugula, asparagus, beets, bell pepper, bok choy, broccoli, brussel sprouts, cabbage, carrots, cauliflower, celery, hot peppers, eggplant, endive, green beans, kale, leeks, lettuce, onion, parsley, peas, spinach, sprouts, turnips, and watercress.

The vegetables to avoid are cucumber, mushrooms, pumpkin, tomatoes, certain varieties of squash (butternut, acorn, and spaghetti), and zucchini.

Kapha and Fruit

For kapha, favor apples, apricots, berries, peaches, pears, pomegranates, prunes, raisins, and occasionally strawberries. Avoid avocado, bananas, coconut, grapefruit, kiwi, oranges, pineapple, plumbs, rhubarb, and watermelon.

Fruit is best eaten in moderation and not paired with other foods. If you're going to have fruit, give your body an hour to digest it before having other foods. And remember that you want to help heat up your digestive fire, so if you're eating fruit it would be helpful to cook it or make sure it's at room temperature (not cold).

Nuts, Seeds, and Condiments for Kapha

Nuts aren't great for kapha, although sometimes having soaked and peeled almonds will be all right. Sprinkling seeds such as chia, flax, poppy, pumpkin, sesame, and sunflower are all right for kapha.

Other things you could add to dishes for some flavor and heat are condiments such as black pepper, cayenne pepper, horseradish, lime juice, mustard, parsley, scallions, sprouts, and wasabi. Some seaweed will be okay for kapha. You can also use rock and sea salt sparingly. Honey is also fine for kapha, in moderation.

QUOTE

> Honey has decongestant, expectorant, and nutritive properties. It helps clear the head, mind, and senses. It is a good vehicle to take with pungent or spicy nervines like bayberry, calamus, ginger, or pippali. —Dr. David Frawley in *Ayurveda and the Mind*

Kapha is sweet, so you don't need more sweet taste in your diet. However, sometimes you will want sweetness. At those times, the best sweetener for kapha is honey. Maple syrup is okay. Try to avoid brown and white sugar, fructose, molasses, and all sugar substitutes.

Dilute Fruit Drinks

It's best to dilute fruit juices for kapha and make sure they are not cooler than room temperature. Fruit juices to try are apple, apricot, berry, cherry, cranberry, and pomegranate. Combining these juices is another possibility: this way you can add creativity and variety to your diet.

Fruit juice isn't the only juice that supports kapha. Vegetable juices are great for kapha, too: mixed vegetable juices and plain carrot juice are especially supportive for kapha types.

Hot Drinks for Kapha

To combat the coolness of kapha, hot drinks can be warming and beneficial for digestion. Make hot drinks out of items from this list: cinnamon, cloves, dandelion, dried ginger, eucalyptus, jasmine, lavender, nettle, peppermint, raspberry, spearmint, and yerba mate. Although hot drinks are helpful for kapha's digestion, avoid caffeinated beverages: caffeine is not supportive to kapha types.

Aromas to Balance Kapha

You'll want to go for what is stimulating and warming when you want to balance kapha. Avoid aromas that are sweet or cooling. Aromas to try in diffusers and oils for kapha are camphor, musk, myrrh, and sage. In cooking, these aromas can help kapha: cinnamon, thyme, basil, and rosemary.

Remember that the best oil to use as a base oil for kapha is corn oil. Because kaphas don't necessarily need more oil on the body or in a bath, you could skip the oil altogether and use a diffuser when you want to use aromatherapy. Another alternative to using a diffuser is to burn sage in a bunch—sage is often bound together to be used for smudging, so it's already bound together for you.

Yoga for Kapha Pacification

Janna Delgado, yoga and Ayurvedic specialist at Kripalu Center for Yoga & Health instructs, "Kaphas should practice in an energetic way, putting in their full effort and pushing beyond their comfort zone." Janna uses the following yoga and breathwork flows to help kaphas focus on coordinating breath with movement to build heat, circulate energy, and fire up metabolism. The flows will also open up the heart, chest, and lungs—all the places where kapha tends to accumulate.

Warm-Up: Sun Salutation

Come into standing, with a tall spine and your feet hip-width apart. Bring your awareness to your breath. Seal your lips and breathe slowly through your nostrils. Work to stabilize and smooth out your breath. Once you have established a steady rhythm, begin strengthening your exhalations by slowly drawing your navel back toward your spine as you breathe out. This abdominal contraction on exhalation will help establish inner heat to melt away excess kapha. Unless otherwise noted, breathe this way throughout the following warm-up and yoga sequence.

The Sun Salutation is a fantastic way to get kapha types moving and warm themselves up. The twelve postures in the sequence effectively stretch, strengthen, and massage all of the joints, muscles, and internal organs of the body. Other benefits include nourishing and balancing the endocrine, circulatory, respiratory, digestive, and immune systems. Move slowly through the sequence, with a focus on deep and steady breathing, to stoke inner heat.

SUN SALUTATION

1. Stand in Mountain Pose with feet hip-width apart and parallel. Distribute the weight evenly between the balls and heels of each foot. Engage the legs and lengthen the spine. Stand tall with relaxed shoulders. Bring your palms together in front of the heart. Notice your breath. Begin taking slow, deep breaths. Use this breath to establish a steady rhythm for the sequence.
2. Inhale and raise the arms out to the sides and up overhead. Press down through the feet, lift out of the waist, and lengthen the fingertips to the sky.
3. Exhale and swan dive forward, sweeping the arms out to the sides as you hinge forward from the hips coming into a Standing Forward Fold.

Place your hands on the floor or your shins. If the hamstrings are tight, bend the knees a bit or use blocks as props underneath your hands.

4. Inhale, press down through the hands and feet, look forward, and lengthen the spine, lifting up halfway into a jackknife position.

5. Exhale and return to Standing Forward Fold, gently drawing the torso toward the thighs.

6. Bend the knees and bring the palms to the floor, framing the feet.

7. Inhale and step the left foot back into a lunge. Sweep the arms forward and overhead for Warrior I. The heart lifts while the shoulders and hips sink into gravity. You may wish to place the left knee on the floor to modify lunge.

8. Exhale, sweep the palms down to the floor to frame the foot, and step the right foot back into Plank Pose, or push-up position. Breathe. To modify, bring the knees to the floor.

9. Exhale and lower to the earth, landing the hips, ribs, and chest all at the same time. Elbows stay close by the sides, fingers spread wide.

10. Plant the palms and pubic bone. Inhale and peel the forehead, chin, and chest away from the earth. Keep the elbows in toward the ribs and the shoulders relaxed.

11. Exhale, curl the toes under, press palms into the ground, and lift the hips toward the sky, coming into Downward Facing Dog. Breathe deeply in this pose. Press the belly and chest back toward the thighs. Lengthen the spine from the crown of the head through the tip of the tailbone. Relax the shoulder blades down the back. Root the palms and heels down. If this pose is too strenuous, come into Table Pose on hands and knees.

12. Inhale and step the left foot between the hands for lunge. You may need to reach back and help the foot step all the way forward. Arms sweep forward and overhead for Warrior I. Lift up through the chest and the crown. Let the shoulders and tailbone relax down. To modify lunge, simply lower the right knee to the floor.

13. Exhale and sweep the hands to the floor, step the right foot beside the left, coming into Standing Forward Fold. Place the hands alongside the feet or on the shins.

14. Inhale and look up as you lift the chest and straighten the arms and legs, coming into jackknife. Root down through the palms and feet. Keep a long spine.

15. Exhale and release back down into Standing Forward Fold. Gently press the belly toward the thighs and the heart toward the shins. Bend the knees slightly if you need to.
16. Ground through the feet and legs. Inhale and sweep the arms out to the sides and overhead as you press all the way up to standing. Palms touch overhead.
17. Exhale and lower the palms down to the heart. Pause.
18. Repeat the sequence once more, leading with the right leg this time. Don't be afraid to break a sweat and challenge yourself!
19. Pause and relax. With your awareness, follow the flow of your breath, letting it gradually slow down. Tune in to the flow of energy throughout your body and mind.

Standing Spinal Twist

Because this rhythmic standing twist focuses on twisting the upper spine (while the hips remain stationary), it is a great way to massage and energize the heart and lungs, break up stagnation in the chest, and rebalance the nervous system. Those with spinal issues such as herniated disc or sacroiliac problems should avoid this pose.

STANDING SPINAL TWIST

1. Stand with your feet parallel, shoulder-width apart. Relax your arms by your sides. Soften your knees.
2. Exhale as you slowly draw your navel back toward your spine and rotate from the waist, turning your rib cage and shoulders to the left. Keep your pelvis stationary and feet flat on the floor. As you do this, bend your elbows and bring your right hand to your left shoulder and your left arm behind your back. Look over your left shoulder.
3. Inhale and sweep through center.
4. Exhale and twist to the right side. Let your arms be soft and relaxed as you twist so one hand taps the front of your shoulder and the back of the other taps your lower back.
5. Create a steady rhythm as you rotate from side to side, coordinating your breath with your movement. Keep your spine relaxed and tall as

you move. Stay focused on strong exhalations and pick up the pace to a comfortable, steady pace.

6. After ten to thirty repetitions, gradually slow the movement down until you return to stillness.

7. Pause and relax for a few breaths. Direct your awareness inside to observe and absorb the effects of the twist.

Angel Breaths

Angel Breaths stimulate and tone the heart, diaphragm, and abdominal organs—all of the places that kapha likes to hang out. Those who suffer from headaches, insomnia, high or low blood pressure, destabilized knees, or sacroiliac or lower back problems should avoid this pose.

1. Reestablish slow and deep breaths through your nostrils.

2. Begin to strengthen your exhalations by slowly contracting your abdominal muscles as you exhale. Do this without strain so the breath stays smooth.

3. Once you have comfortably established breathing with strong exhalations, add a brief pause at the end of each exhalation—just for a second or two—before starting your next inhalation. This technique stokes inner heat and stimulates metabolism.

4. Take a minute to establish this pattern of pausing for a moment at the end of each exhale.

5. Make sure it's sustainable and you are not forcing or straining in any way. Use this breathing pattern throughout this next sequence.

6. Stand with your feet parallel, hip-width apart. Spread your toes wide and press firmly down through the soles of your feet.

7. Release your tailbone down while lifting your sternum and the crown of your head up.

8. Stand tall with your palms together at the center of your chest. Allow your shoulders to relax. Soften the muscles in the face, shoulders, and belly.

9. With your palms still touching, inhale your hands up and overhead.

10. Exhale your arms out to the sides and down as your knees bend and your hips hinge, coming into a squat (deep or shallow, whichever feels best).

11. Palms touch when you reach the bottom of the squat. Pause for a moment or two, suspending your breath, keeping your abdominals engaged.
12. Shift your weight back into your heels as you sink your hips down and lengthen your sternum up.
13. Inhale your hands up the centerline as your legs straighten and your arms reach overhead.
14. Exhale your arms out to the sides and down as your knees and hips bend, sinking into a squat. Palms touch. Pause with your breath held out and your belly engaged.
15. Inhale and draw your palms up the centerline, straightening your legs as your arms lift overhead.
16. Repeat, flowing with your breath—exhaling down into the squat, pausing with breath suspended, inhaling up to standing. The movement of the arms and legs will circulate energy.
17. Continue for five to ten rounds. Then release the movement and become still.
18. Let go of the breathing technique and breathe normally as you absorb the aftereffects of the pose.

Revolved Chair Pose

This pose releases heaviness and dullness, increases flexibility in the spine, and stimulates digestive fire. Those who are pregnant or have spinal issues such as herniated disc or sacroiliac problems should avoid this pose. Those with shoulder, hip, or knee problems should practice this pose gently.

This pose builds on the beginning of the sequence established in Angel Breaths by adding a twist.

1. Stand with your feet together so your toes and heels are touching.
2. Lift your toes and spread them wide. Press your feet firmly into the floor and stand tall.
3. Establish the same breathing patterns as before—long, strong exhalations with a brief suspension of your breath at the bottom of each exhalation. This will establish inner heat and provide a focal point for your mind. Take a moment to establish this breath. Inhale and come into a squat, bending at your knees and hips as you simultaneously lift your arms up alongside your ears with palms touching overhead.

4. On one long, strong exhale, twist your torso and arms to the right, lowering your arms to place your left elbow on the outside of your right knee, then bending your elbows to bring your palms to prayer position at the center of your chest. Pause briefly with the breath held out, drawing your navel toward your spine and leveraging your elbow against your leg to open your chest.
5. Gaze either up at the ceiling or down at your toes.
6. Inhale your arms up and overhead as you unwind and return back to the starting position.
7. Repeat the twist on the other side.
8. Exhale and twist to the left, placing your right elbow on the outside of your left knee, bringing the hands to prayer position at the center of your chest. Pause for a second or two with your breath held out, pressing your right elbow into your left knee to deepen into the twist.
9. Inhale back to center.
10. Synchronize your breath with your movement so you exhale into the twist, pause, and inhale out of the twist. Challenge yourself. Use the retention of the breath to deepen into the twist.
11. Repeat three to five times on each side. Then return to standing.
12. Breathe naturally. Let go of any effort and simply observe the effects of the pose for a few moments.

Rhythmic Forward Fold

This pose will increase enthusiasm, improve digestion, and aid elimination by massaging and stimulating the abdominal organs, reducing your appetite, and expelling excess mucus via the force of gravity. Those who have uncontrolled high blood pressure or are pregnant or those with spinal issues such as herniated disc or sacroiliac problems should avoid this pose.

1. Stand with your feet parallel, hip-width apart.
2. Balance your weight evenly on your feet and firm them into the floor.
3. Stand tall by lifting the crown of your head up toward the ceiling. Inhale and float your arms up and overhead, with palms turned in and fingers reaching up.

4. Exhale and draw your navel in and up as you fold forward from the hips, letting your knees bend slightly and your arms sweep down toward the floor and behind you.
5. Ground through your heels and lift your sitting bones toward the ceiling.
6. On an inhale, sweep back up to standing as you lengthen the front of your torso, reaching your arms up and overhead.
7. Repeat the movement five to ten times.
8. Create a steady rhythm as you move with your breath, contracting your abdominals each time that you fold forward. Then return to standing.
9. Pause and take several breaths in stillness, feeling energy circulating through your body.

Reverse Table

This pose stimulates upward movement of energy to clear the lungs. It also stretches the entire front of the body to increase the flow of energy. Avoid this pose if you have wrist, shoulder, or neck issues.

REVERSE TABLE

1. For this pose, return to the breathing pattern of strong, long exhalations, pausing for a moment or two at the end of each exhale.
2. Sit on the floor with your knees bent, feet hip-distance apart and flat on the floor. Position your heels 12 inches away from your buttocks. Press your palms to the floor behind your hips, shoulder-width apart.
3. With your fingers spread wide, tuck your chin toward your chest. Draw your shoulders back and lift your chest as you inhale deeply.
4. On a long exhalation, press into your feet and hands and lift your hips, thighs, and torso parallel to the floor.
5. Pause with your breath held out for a moment as you draw your navel in toward your spine and up toward your heart. Keep the hips lifted and the chest open.
6. On an inhalation release your buttocks to the floor. Repeat five to ten times, then release the pose and pause for several breaths.

Cooldown

Mellow kaphas will be happy to hear that savasana, or Corpse Pose, is one of the most important postures. It's where the real integration and rebalancing of the doshas takes place. To practice, lie faceup on the floor with your arms and legs extended and your palms facing up. Allow yourself to release tension and completely relax. Let go of everything, including control of the breath. Imagine your body can breathe itself. Enjoy Corpse Pose for five to fifteen minutes, longer if you have time.

Breathwork for Kapha

There are important general guidelines for practicing breath control, pranayama. Review this checklist every time you are going to practice pranayama.

- ❏ Pranayama should be practiced in a quiet, clean, and tranquil location with good ventilation.
- ❏ Pranayama should be practiced on an empty stomach.
- ❏ Pranayama should be done in a comfortable position, either on the floor or in a chair, with the spine, neck, and head erect. Clothing should be loose and comfortable. (Sometimes you may do pranayama while already in another yoga posture if you are already experienced with pranayama.)
- ❏ Avoid strain with all pranayama practices. Do not practice pranayama during times of illness. If you experience negative side effects, physical or emotional, discontinue the practice and consult with a qualified yoga teacher or a physician.

Victorious Breath (Ujjayi)

Victorious Breath has a heating effect that brings lightness and warmth to kapha types. This heat stokes metabolism and digestion and also helps melt excess mucus in the respiratory tract. Those who suffer from respiratory infection, cold, flu, or sore throat or those recovering from recent surgery to the respiratory system should avoid this pranayama.

Victorious Breath is known for the soft hissing sound that is made in the back of the throat during your inhalation and exhalation. By gently constricting the epiglottis—the swallowing muscles in the throat—you create a soft, meditative sound. To begin, sit in a comfortable position with your spine erect. Take a moment to relax your body and tune in to your breath. Notice your breath flowing in and out of your nostrils and allow it to become smooth and rhythmic.

Inhale through your nose, then open your mouth and exhale as you whisper "HAAA." Close the mouth and inhale, slow and deep, through the nose. Repeat this several times, drawing out your exhalation. Then close your mouth and continue to create the HAAA sound from the back of your throat each time you exhale.

Once the sound feels steady and comfortable on the exhalation, try to create the HAAA sound as you inhale by keeping the epiglottis gently constricted. Keep the mouth closed and be careful not to overly constrict your throat. Create the soft HAAA sound on both the inhalation and exhalation. Listen to the sound of the breath and allow it to be smooth and even.

Practice for three to five minutes, gradually increasing your time to seven to ten minutes. Release the pranayama and return to your natural breath. Pause for a few minutes to observe the effects.

Lion's Breath (Simhasana)

Lion's Breath prevents kapha accumulation in the body by stimulating the nerves, senses, and mind. It energizes the immune system, which can get sluggish for kapha types. It also relieves tension in the chest and strengthens the lungs, which are the home of kapha in the body. Avoid this breath if you have recent or chronic injury to the knees, face, neck, or tongue.

LION'S BREATH

1. Sit in a comfortable position, either in a chair or kneeling on the floor with your hips on your heels. Ground your weight down into both sitting bones and reach the crown of the head up to lengthen the spine. Take a moment to relax your body.
2. Close your mouth and notice your breath flowing in and out of your nostrils. Allow it to become steady and rhythmic.

3. Place your hands on your thighs with your fingers fanned out.
4. Inhale deeply through your nose as you draw your belly inward and press your chest forward, arching your upper back. Lift your chin, open your eyes wide, and gaze upward at the spot between the eyebrows.
5. Open your mouth and stick out your tongue. Stretch the tip of your tongue down toward the chin, contract the epiglottis in the front of your throat (the swallowing muscles), and slowly exhale all of the breath out, while whispering a loud, strong "HAAAA" sound.
6. Repeat steps 4 and 5 four to six times. Then pause and relax. Close your eyes and let go as you feel the energy flowing through your head, eyes, throat, and belly.

Skull-Shining Breath (Kapalabhati)

This is an energizing breath that cleanses the lungs and entire respiratory tract. Skull-Shining Breath improves digestion and metabolism, strengthens the abdominal muscles, and energizes the mind.

Because this is such a powerful pranayama, there are several contra-indications. Do not practice this technique if you have any of the following conditions: pregnancy; heart conditions, including hypertension; respiratory conditions; nervous system conditions; recent surgery; inflammation in the abdominal or thoracic regions; or menstruation (the first few days).

Skull-Shining Breath is done by quickly and gently contracting the abdominal muscles during your exhalation and completely relaxing them during your inhalation. This results in a rhythmic pumping of the belly by alternating short, explosive exhales (expulsions) with slightly longer, and passive, inhales. The expulsions force the air out of the lungs—creating a vacuum. The release of the abdominal muscles allows for an automatic inhale to occur as the air sucks back into the lungs to fill the vacuum.

SKULL-SHINING BREATH

1. Sit in a comfortable position with your spine erect. Take a moment to relax your body and tune in to your breath.
2. Seal your lips, and notice your breath flowing in and out of your nostrils. Allow your breath to become steady and deep. You will be breathing through the nostrils throughout this practice.

3. Place one hand on your lower belly to help focus your attention on isolating and contracting this area.
4. Quickly contract your abdominal muscles, pushing a burst of air out of your lungs. Then release the contraction so the belly relaxes, and allow air to passively suck back into your lungs.
5. As you repeat this, let your pace be slow and steady. Repeat fifteen times, creating a comfortable and smooth rhythm. With practice you will become more adept at contracting and releasing your belly.
6. Do one round of fifteen to thirty expulsions to start. Gradually increase to three rounds of thirty expulsions. Allow yourself to take several natural breaths in between each round to integrate the energy of the pranayama.

Integration

When finished with your pranayama practice, return to normal breathing for a minute or two, then lie down in savasana (Corpse Pose) for several minutes to allow for integration.

CHAPTER 13

Stocking the Kitchen

If Ayurvedic cooking is new to you, you may not have the usual go-to ingredients in your kitchen. Once you have the basics on hand, however, you'll have all you need at your fingertips to make meals that will be delicious and balancing for all types. Specific spices, herbs, and oils are key ingredients to keep in the cupboard so you can tailor meals. You will use the staples both in everyday meals and as support if you are noticing imbalance, e.g., if you catch a cold, have mild digestive issues, or can't fall asleep.

Spices and Herbs

The wisdom of Ayurveda explains how to use spices and herbs both as delicious components of a meal and as a necessary means to health and longevity. There are certain spices and herbs to have on hand so you can reach for them both to season your meals and to help ameliorate the beginning symptoms of doshic imbalance.

The following are the typical herbs and spices you will reach for again and again.

- ❑ Basil
- ❑ Black pepper
- ❑ Cardamom
- ❑ Cinnamon
- ❑ Clove
- ❑ Coriander
- ❑ Cumin
- ❑ Fennel
- ❑ Ginger
- ❑ Mint leaves
- ❑ Nutmeg
- ❑ Raw sugar
- ❑ Sea salt
- ❑ Thyme
- ❑ Turmeric

These are the spices that you'll be using often in your cooking. Depending on which doshas you are working to balance and what your tastes are, you may favor some of these spices more than others. You may also favor some more than others depending on the season. Having this variety available makes cooking easy. This way, you'll be able to just reach for different spices as you need them without having to keep running to the store as seasons change and as your vikruti shifts.

FACT

Be mindful when you handle turmeric—it stains most surfaces. If you drip some onto a surface, wipe it immediately with a damp sponge. It may stain your sponges, too. Sometimes you can get a turmeric stain off a surface by using a gentle cleanser, such as Mrs. Meyer's Clean Day Lemon Verbena surface scrub (see *www .mrsmeyers.com*).

Knowing which spices to have available helps you stay stocked and prepared for a wide variety of recipes. Of course, you can add more and make your own spice mixes, too. The above list is simply a list of the basics to start with. You can add from here, or if you never stray much from these, that's okay, too.

Buying, Grinding, and Mixing Spices

If you buy your spices whole, you can use a mortar and pestle to grind them and mix them with other spices. When you grind the spices this way, as you use your own muscle power, be consciously aware of putting healing and loving energy into the spices with every stroke. Another option for grinding whole spices is to use an electric spice grinder.

ESSENTIAL

When you grind spices before cooking, you may want to grind more than you'll use in that one meal. Save the extra so you'll have it ready for the next few meals that will use those spices. That way, you won't need to take time to grind your spices every time you cook.

When using spices in most recipes, you'll want the spices to be in fine powder form. The benefit of a mortar and pestle is that you get a stronger sense of connection to the food through the grinding process. An electric grinder will do well, too: it's a quick and efficient option for creating fine powder.

Where to Get Spices

Most of the spices and herbs that you'll need are available in grocery stores. Dry spices will typically be in the spice aisle, in glass jars. If you buy spices fresh, they may be in a refrigerated section. You can also buy spices online. Some sites to search are:

- Banyan Botanicals: *www.banyanbotanicals.com*
- Penzey's: *www.penzeys.com*

- Dean and Deluca: *www.deandeluca.com*
- The Spice House: *www.thespicehouse.com*

Buy the freshest and highest quality spices that you can afford.

How to Store Spices

Store your spices in airtight glass or plastic containers. Keep them in a cool place: in a drawer or cabinet (out of the sunlight). Also, label the contents of each container clearly, and put the date on the label, too. Your spices will stay fresh enough for about six months to one year. If you have your spices for more than one year, it's time to get fresh spices. Spices are so integral to your cooking that you'll likely use your spices before they go bad.

Whole Foods

Fresh whole foods that don't need to be refrigerated (such as grains, legumes, and seeds) can be kept in airtight containers out of the sunlight for six months to a year. Many grocery stores (usually the ones that have the words *market* or *co-op* in their names) will sell food in bulk. This is a great way to stock up. You can get as much as you think you'll need for a while, and store your items in your reusable containers at home.

Dry Legumes to Keep Stocked

Legumes are one of the main ways you'll be getting your protein. Before you cook legumes, be sure to rinse them a couple of times and pick out any debris or foreign particles. It will be easier to cook and digest some legumes if you soak them first for a few hours. Here are some staple legumes for you to have available:

- ❏ Red lentils
- ❏ Brown or black lentils
- ❏ Mung dahl
- ❏ Aduki beans
- ❏ Black beans
- ❏ Split peas
- ❏ Chickpeas

Legumes are such a good part of any meal because you can doctor them up with spices, mix them with rice, and/or add vegetables to them. You can prepare them like a stew on cold nights, or make lighter recipes other times of the year and use them as side dishes or appetizers (e.g., hummus or bean dip).

Grains

Grains are an important part of your diet. They provide you with a variety of nutrients and can be seasoned to be either sweet or savory, depending on your tastes and what your body's needs are. Also, some are gluten free. Amaranth, millet, and quinoa, for example, are gluten free and provide you with a good dose of protein to boot!

ESSENTIAL

In addition to important vitamins, minerals, and healthy fats, whole grains provide a good dose of fiber. Among its many attributes, fiber helps prevent constipation, thus supporting the body in elimination. Some high-fiber grains are amaranth, brown rice, buckwheat, millet, quinoa, spelt, whole rye, steel-cut oats and rolled oats (even instant oatmeal), and whole wheat couscous.

While Western culture focuses so much on the nutrients of foods, Ayurveda honors food for its healing potential that goes beyond nutritive value. Remember that these grains grow because of the energy of the natural elements, and thus they carry the life-force energy of all of the elements within them. Those very elements help the seeds to grow, and that energy will be transferred to you when you eat your meal.

Maya Tiwari, in her book *Living Ahimsa Diet: Nourishing Love & Life*, writes, "We must begin to see all plants and the ahimsa (nonviolent) practices that sustain them as reaching as far as the galaxies and stars. These practices are not only about composting, sowing, and then reaping the bounty of nature, they are also about recognizing the divine life carried by each seed and grain, life they give to us as sustenance and memory."

By taking time to remember that there is natural and sustaining life-force in each grain, you open yourself up to taking in that energy. Without cultivating this awareness, you aren't receiving all the potential energy that your food has to offer—energy that is life-sustaining for you.

It's so easy to find ways to put whole grains into your diet. Whole grains are incredibly versatile. You can eat them as breakfast cereal, as part of a lunch burrito or midday salad, or mixed together with vegetables or legumes for dinner. Here is a list of grains to have in your cupboard:

❑ Amaranth
❑ Millet
❑ Whole oats
❑ Quinoa
❑ Basmati rice
❑ Brown rice

Experiment with grains and find out which textures and recipes you like best. If some of these grains are new to you and you don't like the first recipe you try, keep in mind that you may like the grain in a different recipe. Because they can be used in so many ways, grains taste differently based on what foods and spices you prepare them with. It might take you a couple of tries before you find your favorite ways to enjoy the various grains.

Nuts and Seeds

Nuts and seeds are wonderful to be used as a snack or as a part of your meal. Which nuts and seeds you choose will depend on your constitution. See Table 13.1.

▼ **13.1: NUTS AND SEEDS TO FAVOR**

Dosha	Nuts	Seeds
Vata	almonds, black walnuts, Brazil nuts, cashews, charole, coconut, filberts, hazelnuts, macadamia nuts, peanuts, pecans, pine nuts, pistachios, walnuts	chia, flax, halva, pumpkin, sesame, sunflower, tahini
Pitta	almonds (soaked and peeled), charole, coconut	flax, halva, popcorn (buttered, no salt), psyllium, pumpkin, sunflower
Kapha	charole	chia, flax, popcorn (buttered, no salt), pumpkin, sunflower

From *The Complete Book of Ayurvedic Home Remedies* by Dr. Vasant Lad

As always, if you find that a certain nut or seed isn't working for you, stop eating it and let your specialists and doctors know.

Ghee and Oils

Ghee and oils are very nourishing, supportive, and balancing. Keep the oils stocked that are most needed for you and your family, based on constitution.

Oils for Vata Types

Vatas do well with a lot of oil. To combat the dry and cool qualities, keep sesame oil stocked for self-massage.

At meals, vatas can put a healthy helping of ghee in their food. Use it to sauté or cook with instead of butter, and drop half a tablespoon into your dish when the food is piping hot and ready to eat. Ghee can be used in most anything from grains to vegetables to legumes.

Olive oil and sesame oil are the two oils to favor when cooking for vata. Most oils will work well for vata; however, avoid coconut oil when preparing food for vata.

Oils for Pitta

Pitta does well with most oils. As is the case with vata, ghee can be used often for pitta. Sunflower oil is the best for pitta. Canola, olive, flaxseed, and walnut oils are also good to cook with for pitta. The best oils for pitta's self-massage are sunflower and coconut.

Oils for Kapha

Kapha doesn't need a lot of extra oil. A bit of oil will be good for kapha, even though kapha is already moist. Corn, canola, and sesame are the best oils for kapha. Ghee won't harm kapha—ghee is good for all doshas. Olive oil is not a good balancing oil for kapha.

How to Make Ghee

1. Put 1 pound sweet, unsalted butter into a medium-sized pot.

2. On medium heat, melt the butter, without burning it.

3. Allow the butter to boil. Stir occasionally, as the butter boils and sputters a bit.

4. Soon you'll notice the ghee becoming a clear golden color and white solid pieces will form. When the bubbling has quieted down, the ghee is ready. This whole process takes about 10–15 minutes.

5. Remove the ghee from the heat immediately. At this stage it's prone to burn.

6. Let the ghee cool slightly.

7. Pour the ghee through cheese cloth or a metal strainer into a clean, glass jar, separating the solids from the clear ghee.

8. Store at room temperature, and when you spoon ghee out, make sure the spoon is clean and dry.

Dressing a Salad

Nuts and oils are great on salads, so use the above guidelines for choosing what would be best to add to yours. Keep in mind that ghee is great for all the doshas, though it should be used in moderation for kapha. Ghee can be used in many foods, but it's not the best choice for salads. For salads, in general, vatas would do well with olive oil, and all the doshas could benefit from sunflower oil.

Some Items to Keep in the Fridge

While spices, oils, and legumes are best kept at room temperature, there will be some items best kept in the fridge. So what should your refrigerator have in it to keep you prepared?

Vegetables, Fruits, and Berries

Get organic, locally grown whole vegetables, fruits, and berries when possible. Buy what is in season, and choose an assortment of foods that naturally come in a variety of colors. Keep in mind, of course, your constitution and the constitution of those for whom you are cooking.

If you don't cook at home every night, it's okay to buy frozen vegetables, fruits, and berries because they will last longer. Read the packages to get what is most fresh, whole, and natural. You don't want added colors or flavorings, for example.

Nut and Seed Butters

Nut butters are versatile. They are perfect on vegetables and fruit. Peanut butter isn't the only nut or seed butter available, though it's very popular in the West. Almond and sunflower butters are also delicious and great options. Choose which nut is best for your constitution, and keep nut butter in the refrigerator once opened.

Natural Sweeteners

Sweet is a great taste for vata and pitta types. Kapha would do well to go lightly with sweets, but all doshas can use all of the six tastes. So, having sweeteners around is good for everyone.

Sweeteners to Stock

Maple syrup and honey are perhaps the most commonly used natural sweeteners in the West. Molasses and rice syrup are other options, too. See Table 13.2 for which sweeteners each dosha should favor.

▼ **13.2: DOSHAS AND SWEETENERS TO FAVOR**

Dosha	Sweetener
Vata	honey, molasses, rice syrup
Pitta	maple syrup, rice syrup
Kapha	honey

Remember that sweet is also one of the six tastes, so you can find sweet in foods without adding sweetener when you're craving the sweet taste.

Teas and Brews

Drinking tea or brews is an important part of your Ayurvedic lifestyle. By drinking teas and brews, you can bring balance to your doshas, energize yourself during the day, and relax yourself before going to bed. There are so many recipes for brews and teas that Ayurveda suggests, and having some ingredients on hand can be helpful for when you need just the right warm drink.

Teas Already Prepared for You

The grocery store has a variety of teas available. Good choices to have on hand are peppermint tea (can ease digestive discomfort and help you relax at bedtime), ginger tea (to support digestion), and tulsi tea (also called "holy basil," used for a variety of health benefits, including helping to give you a boost if you are low on energy).

If you want to try blends that are already packaged for you, the following are some companies to support your quest. You also have the option of making your own blends, simply and with love.

- The brand Traditional Medicinals has a variety of teas made to help support your health: *www.traditionalmedicinals.com*
- Goldthread Herbal Apothecary sells a variety of healing blends packaged loose in 100 percent biodegradable clear cellulose bags: *www.goldthreadapothecary.com*
- Yogi Tea bases its choices of herbs and botanicals on Ayurvedic philosophy: *www.yogiproducts.com*
- Pukka is a UK brand named for its commitment to "authentic" and "genuine" practice and products: *www.pukkaherbs.com*
- Tea Forté sells teas loosely packed in silken pyramid tea bags in unique blends: *www.teaforte.com*
- Rishi Tea sells organic fair trade teas: *www.rishi-tea.com*

- Harney & Sons has paired up with the Chopra Center, creating Ayurvedic-inspired blends, and they have a large assortment of their own, as well: *www.harney.com*

Making Your Own Tea or Brew

To make your own tea you'll need a teapot and either a strainer, a tea infuser, or tea filters (you can buy one made of reusable cloth or those made of biodegradeable paper). Some teapots come with their own strainer or infuser. To use those, put your herbs into the strainer, pour boiling water over it, and let it steep for the desired amount of time. Then, when you pour the tea into your mug, the herbs stay in the strainer. If you don't want to use a strainer, you can buy reusable or biodegradeable tea bags to put your herbs in for individual cups of tea. Teavana sells biodegradeable tea filters: *www .teavana.com/tea-products/tea-makers-infusers/p/perfect-paper-tea-filters*

Some Types of Teas and Brews

You can make your own simple brews by putting your desired herbs in boiling water or warm milk and letting them steep.

As you prepare for bed, make yourself mint tea by putting mint in the tea filter or infuser, pouring boiling water over it, then letting it steep for five to seven minutes before drinking.

QUESTION

How often should I drink tea?
Your specialist may recommend you take brews at specific times in the day, in relationship to when you eat or sleep. What she recommends will depend on how the elements are showing up in you and how your digestive fire is working. At times, she will change the ratio and types of spices depending on what she notices about your health.

Make your own ginger brew by grating two teaspoons of fresh ginger, putting it in the bottom of a mug, then pouring boiling water over it and letting it steep for ten minutes. To add some complexity to the brew, after ten minutes, add two teaspoons of honey and a few squirts of lemon juice. (You could also drink the ginger brew without the honey and lemon.) A great time to drink this brew would be a half hour before a meal to get the digestive fire stimulated.

Cumin, coriander, fennel tea is a common brew to take for helping digestion. You can take this once per day (or as recommended by your specialist) to help remove toxins from the body in a very gentle way. To make this tea, put one teaspoon each of cumin, coriander, and fennel into your strainer or filter, then steep in boiling water for about ten to fifteen minutes. A good time to drink this brew is about a half hour after finishing your meal.

Some herbs are stronger than others, so it's best to talk with your Ayurvedic specialist before experimenting. She can tell you which herbs to take in tea on a regular basis and which to be more cautious about, especially when considering your constitution.

CHAPTER 14

What About . . . ?

In Western culture, you can always find new information circulating about which foods to avoid and the harmful effects those foods will yield. Sometimes it seems that the list of forbidden foods changes as often as you prepare to make a trip to the grocery store. You may wonder what you should avoid and why. You may hear and read conflicting information in the media, so it may be hard for you to decide if there's anything to avoid and why that would be. Ayurveda can help answer these questions.

Sattvic, Rajasic, Tamasic

When thinking about what to eat, you now know it's important to think about the qualities of the food and the qualities of the elements in and around you. You know that for health, you will choose foods with the qualities that are the opposite of the qualities you're feeling and exhibiting. This will create balance in you so your mind and body will be working well and easefully. You also know to think about the qualities of the tastes of the food, not just the qualities of the physical texture and temperature of the food.

There's also another categorization that Ayurveda offers that describes the human temperament. This category is composed of sattvic, rajasic, and tamasic. When talking about food, these qualities are used to describe the effects the food will have on your mental and emotional state.

When it comes to food, here is how you can think of sattvic, rajasic, and tamasic:

- **Sattvic:** fresh, pure, light, and easy to digest
- **Rajasic:** stimulating
- **Tamasic:** heavy, dulling, leading to illness and disorders

These qualities greatly influence your mental state. For example, if you are predominantly vata and sattvic, then the qualities of vata that you'll notice most are your creativity, clear thinking, and lightness. If you are predominantly vata and rajasic, then you will likely feel anxiety, fear, and hyperactivity—the more mobile effects of vata. If you are predominantly vata and tamasic, you could feel sadness, grief, and confusion.

Mental States and Your Constitution

No matter what your constitution, you can use the terms *sattva*, *rajas*, and *tamas* to describe your mental state. Across the board, being sattvic in nature will bring out the healthiest, purest, and most desirable qualities of the elements in you. This doesn't mean you can't ever eat foods that might be rajasic or tamasic in nature. Natural and whole foods from all categories have something to offer. For example, avocadoes are tamasic, and because of their moist and heavy qualities they are a good balance for vata. That being said, vatas can still eat avocadoes in moderation. Too much of anything can create imbalance.

Eating Meat

It's been said that thousands of years ago when Ayurveda began, the sages would recommend eating meat if it was appropriate for a person's health and diet. People hunted animals in their natural environment, killed them in a nontorturous way, and did not pump them with chemicals. Because the animal lived its life in nature and it was killed without having to suffer, the energetic qualities of the meat would have been pure and clean.

It's also been said that vegetarianism has been chosen by many on the Ayurvedic path for centuries. There are those who view killing animals in any way, compassionately or not, as a violation of **ahimsa**, nonviolence. Those who are vegetarians and promote vegetarianism believe that meat is not needed for the sustenance of a human life, and if peace on earth is to prevail then animals must not be killed for food.

Nonviolence and Eating Meat

Nonviolence, ahimsa, is of utmost importance to the Ayurvedic lifestyle (and it's one of the core tenets of a yogic lifestyle). Those who support vegetarianism explain that this means we cannot kill animals for food. Many also say that because animals are treated inhumanely before the meat arrives at markets and grocery stores, eating meat that's been processed this way would not be supported by Ayurvedic specialists today. It's also said that any chemicals or suffering the animal endures in its life or death would not be supportive to your body or mind when you ingest it.

Still, there are plenty of Ayurvedic specialists and nutritionists who recommend having meat in one's diet. If you choose to eat some meat in your diet, here are questions you can ask. This way, you'll be informed about what you're buying and eating.

QUESTIONS TO ASK ABOUT MEAT

- ❏ Where does your meat come from?
- ❏ How are the animals kept and treated?
- ❏ What are the animals fed?
- ❏ How are they killed?
- ❏ How fresh is the meat when you get it?

Answering these questions will help you determine how beneficial it will be for you to eat the beef, chicken, fish, seafood, etc. Local and organic farms are becoming more and more in demand, so hopefully you could find one near you and get the answers you need about what you'll be eating.

QUOTE

> Although I truly believe that a vegetarian diet is the most healthful diet for human beings, in our culture it is extremely difficult, if not impossible, to maintain. Because of this, I don't recommend a vegetarian diet for children. Many vegetarian kids and adults do not maintain a high-enough quality diet; they then become addicted to sugar for their nutritional energy instead of obtaining energy from a well-balanced vegetarian diet. —John Douillard

John Douillard, in *Perfect Health for Kids: Ten Ayurvedic Health Secrets Every Parent Must Know*, warns that it can be difficult in our culture to get the protein the body needs, especially during the winter months. His advice for those who want to be vegetarians is to be diligent about eating well. To do this, eat nuts, seeds, legumes, beans, and whole grains, making sure to get your needed doses of protein. Douillard suggests supplementing the whole foods with dairy and also whey-based protein shakes if you still aren't getting enough protein.

An important question to consider, as you think about your choice whether to eat meat or not, is what nonviolence means to you. And would you like to find ways to get protein from sources other than meat? Your Ayurvedic specialist can help and give you support if you have questions. If you want to be a vegetarian, plenty of information is available. There are many sources of protein that are not meat.

If you don't want to give up meat, when you choose an Ayurvedic specialist, be sure to pick one who supports that choice. There are different preferences out there, and you'll want someone who can support your choices.

Meat as Tamasic

Another thing to consider about meat is that it is tamasic. Tamasic qualities are heavy, dull, and lead to illness. Because of the heavy quality of meat and its high level of protein, when vata is out of balance, a person may turn to meat to help get balanced. Turning to a good source of protein can really help vata feel more in balance. If you are a vegetarian, try avocadoes. Remember that truly, meat isn't the only option.

Dairy

When it comes to dairy, as with all foods, talk to your doctors and specialists. Some people are intolerant of milk, particularly milk that has been chemically treated and processed. In terms of elemental qualities, most dairy products are cooling.

Vata and Dairy

Milk is sattvic, and warm milk can be especially soothing for vata. Sour cream and yogurt are just fine for vata (in moderation), especially because of their sour taste and oily quality.

ESSENTIAL

Even though you store dairy in the refrigerator, it would be best for vata if you would allow the dairy to come to room temperature before eating or drinking it. So, whether it's milk on your cereal, sour cream on your baked potato, or yogurt with granola, allow the dairy to warm up to room temperature before you enjoy it.

Most dairy is balancing for vata. Buy milk that is local, organic, and from a healthy cow. Butter, buttermilk, cow's milk, goat's milk, cheese, yogurt—all are good for countering the effects of vata.

Kapha and Dairy

Dairy and kapha have similar qualities, so it's best for kaphas to be mindful about how much dairy they have in their diet. Kaphas can try buttermilk because of its lightness in contrast to other forms of dairy, such as hard cheeses and ice cream, which are high in fat. Kaphas could also try goat's milk and a little bit of ghee to satisfy a dairy craving.

Ice cream, because it's cold and high in fat, will increase kapha. If you're kapha and you're really craving ice cream in the summertime, when it's not kapha season, that's a great time (seasonally) to have ice cream. Remember that enjoyment of life is very important, and for many people ice cream is synonymous with the inauguration of summer. If taking ice cream completely out of your diet feels like deprivation, don't take it completely out. Also, you could try frozen yogurt, which has less fat.

Pitta and Diary

While vatas would do all right with salted butter, buttermilk, yogurt, sour cream, and hard cheeses, these dairy products would aggravate the fire in pitta. Other than those dairy products, most dairy is fine for pitta. A predominantly pitta type might do very well with the following dairy products, in moderation, in her diet:

- Unsalted butter
- Soft cheese
- Goat's milk
- Cow's milk
- Ghee
- Cottage cheese
- Ice cream

Especially during the summer months and when the sun is high in the sky, pitta is high in the natural world. Having cool and sweet dairy products can help pacify pitta, particularly during the height of pitta season.

Drinking Alcohol

As is the case with other food and drink, you have the ability to observe how alcohol affects you. You don't need a doctor or an Ayurvedic specialist to tell you how alcohol affects you, personally: it's usually rather obvious how well you tolerate different kinds of alcohol and what the effects are. Even so, Ayurveda has wisdom to share about drinking alcohol.

Alcohol Is Tamasic

Alcohol is tamasic, which means it is heavy, dulling, and weakens the body's immune system. You may hear people say they turn to alcohol to "numb" their feelings; that is one way of acknowledging alcohol's "dulling" quality.

ESSENTIAL

If you are addicted to alcohol, talk to your doctor and your Ayurvedic specialist. Ayurvedic wisdom has protocols to help with addictions. Your specialist may first recommend panchakarma, which means "five actions." For panchakarma, you'll perform specific actions to prepare your body for eliminating toxins, and then other actions will help you expel the toxins from your body.

Consumption of too much alcohol can lead to many imbalances, from depression to failing organs. Alcohol is also known to destroy brain cells, reduce bone mass, and cause incontinence.

Alcohol as a Medicinal

In the classic texts of Ayurveda, alcohol was used as medicinal. It is also known to combat fatigue and to stimulate digestion.

Herbal wines can still be prepared and used today to help the body regain health and balance. See Dr. David Frawley's *Ayurvedic Healing* for herbal wine recipes, and of course check in with your Ayurvedic specialist to discuss how certain herbs and wine will likely affect you. Knowing which alocoholic beverages and herbs are good for you can be a very beneficial part of your healthy life.

Good News for Chocolate Lovers

Some chocolate can be good for you, especially raw cacao. Cacao and chocolate aren't the same thing, so understanding the terms will help you understand what you're putting into your body when you reach for chocolate bliss.

Chocolate comes from the cacao bean. The cacao bean matures inside a pod that looks like a football, and grows in the rainforest. Under heavy shade, cacao beans are harvested. To make "chocolate," people process the cacao and add milk and sugar. This makes the cacao bean into the smooth, creamy commercial bars you buy at the supermarket. Because of the added ingredients and processing, the final chocolate product that is mass-produced is very different from what you would experience from eating raw cacao or chocolate that is of very high quality (organic, less processed, and containing fewer refined or artificial added ingredients).

Cacao and Your Health

Naked Chocolate by David Wolfe and Shazzie is an indispensible resource for learning about cacao's history and its many benefits. The story of cacao (including its term in history as a form of currency!), the way people make chocolate, and a selection of recipes in this book can help you incorporate cacao into your diet in a healthy and exciting way.

The cacao bean, like so much in nature, is chockful of nutrients and energy to support the body. It contains a variety of nutritive elements including calcium, dopamine, fiber, iron, magnesium, polyphenols, and protein.

Cacao Brings Bliss

According to Wolfe and Shazzie's research, neuroscientist Daniele Piomelli discovered in 1996 that cacao contains the neurotransmitter anandamide. *Ananda* means "bliss" in Sanskrit, and the word *ananda* comes up often along the path of yoga and Ayurveda. According to ancient yogic philosophy, you have a "bliss" body, which you can tap in to during practices such as yoga and meditation. Spending time connected to your bliss body is healing and rejuvenating for your mind and body. Anandamide is a modern scientific term, derived from the Sanskrit *ananda*.

The pharmacological effects of anandamide indicate that it may play an important part in the regulation of mood, memory, appetite, and pain perception. It may act as the chief component in the control of cognition and emotion. Psychological experiments demonstrate that anandamide may be as important as the more well-known neurotransmitters dopamine and serotonin. —David Wolfe and Shazzie

When you eat cacao, you can be sure there is scientific proof explaining why it helps you feel good, control your appetite, and regulate your mood. As with everything else, of course, it must be taken in moderation and with mindfulness for the best effects.

Keep Dark Chocolate or Cacao in Your Bag

If you buy organic chocolate that is dark, it doesn't contain a lot of added milk and sugar. Dark chocolate has a higher cacao content than milk chocolate. The taste of both dark chocolate and raw cacao is much different from the taste of its milky, sugary, highly processed chocolate counterparts. Because of this, eating dark chocolate is a unique experience.

Cocoa beans and their creation into chocolate have been prized for their health and wellness benefits for hundreds of years. There's magic in this precious food: chocolate is inspiration for the soul. —Joshua Needleman, Chocolate Springs Café

When you eat a milk chocolate bar from a supermarket, it can be addictive and may not satisfy your craving. You may also feel a quick high and then a low drop after eating a milk chocolate bar—that is from the sugar. In the grocery checkout line, you could find yourself gulping down a bagful of mini chocolate candies or wolfing down a candy bar and still not feel as though your craving has been satisfied. This has to do not with the cacao but with the added artificial or refined ingredients.

Cacao pods grow on theobroma cacao trees. *Theobroma* means "food of the gods." The Incas, Mayans, and Aztecs treated cacao as sacred. They made drinks with it for special ceremonies and gave it to their warriors and noblemen for strengthening and healing.

Raw cacao and dark chocolate can be very satisfying in only a few bites. Cacao when raw or in dark chocolate isn't the kind of food that you will feel compelled to keep shoveling into your mouth. It is strong and satisfying in taste, nutrients, and energy. If you like chocolate, carry a high-quality bar of dark chocolate or raw cacao nibs in your bag. You may find that just a few bites daily or every few days could be just what you need from the cacao bean.

How Chocolate Fits into an Ayurvedic Lifestyle

Chocolate is warm, heavy, and moist. Because of these qualities, it's good for vata, and not so helpful to pitta or kapha. It also contains caffeine, which is aggravating to pitta. At the same time, cacao and dark chocolate can have slightly bitter and astringent tastes, which can be balancing for pitta and kapha.

How to Deal with Allergies

When you suffer from allergies, it's disruptive to your life, and it's a signal that your body is in a reactive state. Whether it's food allergies or seasonal allergies, your Ayurvedic specialist can work with you to help minimize the occurrence of allergies and deal with them when they occur.

Eat Well for Your Type

One of the best things you can do to prevent allergies is to eat in a way that keeps your constitution in balance. By keeping your constitution in balance, you are keeping your body healthy and supporting it to perform its purifying functions well. This means that the lymphatic system is doing its job to clear out toxins, your body is digesting and circulating nutrients, and your elimination is easeful and daily (once or twice per day, well-formed, about the size of a banana). When your body is able to eliminate toxins, bacteria, waste, etc., then the allergic symptoms either don't begin or they are short-lived. Eating right is a very important step in this process.

Also, pay attention to which foods cause you to have allergic symptoms. When you notice these symptoms, think about cutting out the foods that create these symptoms in you. Allergic reactions can produce any of these symptoms:

- ❏ Bloating stomach and gas
- ❏ Headache
- ❏ Wheezing
- ❏ Sneezing
- ❏ Hay fever
- ❏ Cold
- ❏ Sinus infection
- ❏ Asthma
- ❏ Rash
- ❏ Itching
- ❏ Hives

Your Ayuredic specialist will determine if your allergies seem to be vata, pitta, or kapha in nature. This will help her determine which herbs and purification methods to recommend to help you rid the body of the irritant and strengthen your immunity.

FACT

Taking triphala at night before bed has a mild laxative effect. It works for all doshas. This will support elimination as you work to clear the body of what is causing your reaction.

If you are vata or pitta, be sure that you are using enough oil in your diet. It's extremely important to keep your body internally lubricated. You can do this by making sure you are using ghee and oils in your meals: choose the type of oil that is right for your type.

Other ways to make sure your body is well-lubricated is to use oil in the nasal passages, practice self-massage daily with oil before taking a shower, and stay hydrated. Drink plenty of water throughout the day—don't wait until you feel thirsty.

If you drink plenty of liquid and make sure you are taking in enough oil, this will help your body stay lubricated internally. Self-massage daily with oil is another practice to begin. When you add this to your daily routine, the oil will penetrate through the skin into tissues and bone.

WHY KEEP THE BODY LUBRICATED TO FIGHT ALLERGIES?

- Ghee or oil in the nasal passages prevents allergens from nestling into mucous membranes in the nose.
- If mucous membranes get dried out, they produce more mucus as a reaction—this could cause too much mucus and lead to congestion, which can then lead to colds, upper respiratory infections, and more serious complications.
- Keeping the body lubricated helps keep the mucous production to just the right level. You have mucous membranes throughout the body. If there's too much mucous production (in reaction to dryness), the mucous can create clogs in your system instead of allowing the mucous to flow freely as it tries to carry bacteria, allergens, and other contaminants out of the body.
- Keeping the body moist supports the lymphatic system, which carries waste and toxins out of the body. If the body gets dried out, the lymphatic system can become sluggish. If the lymphatic system becomes sluggish, toxins build in the body, and then the body becomes more sensitive. This can lead to allergies, colds, viruses, flu, etc.
- A healthy amount of mucus is needed throughout the digestive tract to help food move through. Too little mucus will make the intestines and stomach vulnerable and reactive to acid and spices, and too much mucus will hinder the necessary passage of food through the intestines and stomach.

Elimination of waste is one of the most important ways that you stay healthy. If your body is able to move waste and contaminants out of the body effectively and efficiently, that will directly and significantly contribute to your health and longevity. So stay hydrated, use oils on the body, and make sure your diet has enough oil in it.

Are You Dehydrated?
Some signs of dehydration are:

❑ Headaches
❑ Irritability
❑ Muscle cramps
❑ Fatigue
❑ Constipation
❑ Migraine

Drinking plenty of water could be enough to ameliorate and prevent these symptoms. Of course, if you are having any conditions that are not normal, talk to your doctor and specialists.

The number of ounces of water you should drink daily is your weight (in pounds) divided by two. For example, if you weigh 140 pounds, then you should drink 70 ounces of water per day. Ayurveda recommends that you sip warm water throughout the day rather than gulp down a huge amount of water a few times a day. When you sip water throughout the day, your body can absorb it better. If you drink too much at once, most of it will just run right through your system.

That being said, it's still okay to drink an entire glass first thing in the morning, to drink some water with your meals, and drink full glasses when you want to. Just also be sure to sip throughout the day for the best results. And, always choose warm or room temperature water. Cold water hampers your digestive fire, which helps you digest everything from meals to emotions to experiences.

Meditation, Yoga, and Breathwork

Meditation, yoga, and breathwork for your type can help your health all around. It can also help reduce allergies. Allergies tend to be caused by too much stress on the body. Stress can come in the form of mental stress, environmental stress, physical stress, and a combination of any or all of these.

Stress creates imbalance in the mind and in the body. Regularly including meditation, yoga, and breathwork into your life can reduce stress and thus reduce your body's sensitivity to pollutants and allergens. See Appendix B for a list of guided CDs that can guide you on a practice specifically for your dosha.

CHAPTER 15

Natural Remedies

Ayurveda has natural remedies for common symptoms. The common symptoms are considered early signs of imbalance, so it's great for you to prevent them or catch them early. They include seasonal allergies, colds, gas, bloating, headaches, lower back pain, insomnia, and more. It's always best to talk to your Ayurvedic specialist and doctor when you notice these symptoms so you can both determine root causes and rule out more serious conditions. The following are some remedies Ayurveda recommends, and you can make them easily at home.

For Colds

When you notice a cold coming on, start to support your body in clearing out the mucus and irritants. Be sure you are hydrating yourself well, and get extra rest. One way to prevent colds is to keep your immune system strong by keeping yourself balanced as best you can. Then you will either avoid catching colds altogether, or when you do catch one it will be much easier to treat.

Turmeric for Colds

Turmeric is an anti-inflammatory that will also clear excess mucous (for children and adults alike). One way to take turmeric is to make a paste of equal parts turmeric and raw honey. Begin by taking one tablespoon of this mixture every hour for the first few hours, and then reduce the frequency to once about every four to six hours. If symptoms do not improve after the first day, talk to your doctor.

FACT

Children over two years of age typically can take this remedy, too, with a smaller dosage. The dosage for children should be one teaspoon at a time.

You can also add turmeric to your diet on a regular basis, and not wait until you catch a cold. It's a delicious seasoning to add to rice, pasta, and vegetables any time of year. For a more complex taste, mix it with other spices to create a curry powder.

Ginger for Colds and Flu

An excellent ingredient for combating a cold or flu is ginger. The extra mucus your body creates comes from excess kapha, and it's possible that vata will be in excess as well when you have a cold or flu—leading to chills and poor appetite.

ESSENTIAL

Dr. Lad warns not to take aspirin and ginger at the same time; they both thin the blood. Take them at least two hours apart if you want to take them both. Because of the dangers of improper food, herb, and medicine combining, get advice from your specialist before trying remedies at home that are new to you.

Ginger is hot, pungent, and stimulating, which is great for countering the effects of too much kapha and vata. In *Ayurvedic Home Remedies*, Dr. Lad gives a simple recipe for a ginger brew to take several times a day when you have a cold or flu:

Ginger Brew

1. Combine ginger, cinnamon, and lemongrass in the ratio 1:1:2, or substitute a pinch of cardamom for the lemongrass.

2. Steep this mixture in hot water for ten minutes, then strain.

3. If you'd like to add sweetness, use honey.

You can make an even simpler brew by steeping only freshly grated ginger in boiling water. After about ten minutes, drink and savor the healing effects of ginger.

Steaming

Steaming is a fast and effective way to deal with congestion, sore throat, and runny nose. You can simply pour boiling water into a bowl, then hold your head over the bowl with a towel over your head to keep the steam in. Close your eyes and breathe deeply.

Spend about ten to fifteen minutes inhaling the steam. You can do this several times a day.

You can steam with plain water, or add a drop of eucalyptus essential oil or tea tree essential oil to the bowl after you've poured the boiling water into it. These herbs are naturally antiseptic. Inhale the steam nice and deeply into the sinuses, back of the throat, and lungs.

For Gas

Gas is common and is often due to excess air in the colon. When you have gas, allow yourself to release it from the body as flatulence or burping. Gas in the colon is considered an excess of vata, and holding it in will create more vata disturbance in the body.

Pacify Vata

If you're feeling the pain of gas in the colon often, and you have a lot of flatulence, try a vata-pacifying diet. This will help bring moisture and heaviness into your body, to balance the winds of vata.

Also, when you perform your daily self-massage, make sure you are oiling your torso well. Gently massage the area of your torso where the colon is, bringing your awareness and care to that area of the body, back and front.

Regulate Your Elimination

Sometimes gas builds up in conjunction with constipation, another sign of vata imbalance. You can regulate your elimination by taking triphala. Triphala is available in tablets and in powder. Take a tablet with a glass of water, or boil a teaspoon of the powdered form in water. Take triphala before going to bed. It's a mild herb, suitable for all doshas, so you can take it regularly, for four to six weeks.

A Mixture to Take after Meals

Roast cumin, coriander, and ajwan seeds, in equal parts. To do this, roast each type of seed separately in a dry pan. While roasting, which should take one to three minutes, stir the seeds often to prevent burning. Once they are roasted, remove them from the heat. Mix all the seeds together, and carry the mixture with you throughout your day. After each meal, put about a teaspoon of the mixture in your mouth, chew it well, then wash it down with a few mouthfuls of warm water.

Another option to help digestion is to make a ginger tea. You can sip the tea on an empty stomach or drink it about a half hour before meals to help get the digestive fire going.

For Lower Back Pain

Low back pain can be caused by several factors, emotional as well as physical. Certain home remedies can help, though serious injuries (like a slipped disc) will require professional medical attention and supervision.

Remedies for Lower Back Pain

When you have lower back pain, or any back pain, your Ayurvedic specialist may recommend certain herbs to help relax the muscles. You also can rub mahanarayan oil on the affected area and take a hot bath, or lie down in a comfortable position and try this visualization:

1. Lie down in a comfortable position. If you're on your back, place a pillow or two underneath your knees. If you're curled up on your side, place a pillow in between your knees. See if those pillows make the posture more comfortable.
2. Envision the muscles of the back relaxing into the support of the floor beneath you.
3. Take deep nourishing breaths; on each inhale envision your breath carrying healing life-force energy to the entire back, especially the area that hurts.
4. On each exhale, envision exhaling any pain, emotional and physical.
5. After several rounds of deep breaths, return to normal breathing. Envision relaxing the entire body.

When you're ready to sit up after this visualization, sit up very slowly. There's no rush.

Visualizations are very powerful healing tools. When you're experiencing any kind of pain in the body, visualize health and comfort where you feel pain. Place your hand on that body part, too, if you can reach it. The visualization will let your body know you are responding to its "alarm signal," which is what pain is.

The benefits of learning to relax and let go cannot be overstated. Your mind and body need time to restore, relax, and rejuvenate. Stress is often cited as the cause of imbalance and illness. Practice letting it all go.

Pacify Vata

Because the colon is located in the same region of the body as the lower back, disturbances in vata can cause low back pain. If you experience lower back pain, follow a vata-pacifying diet, keep yourself warm, surround yourself with calming friends and family, and create routine when you can—at the very least, at mealtimes and bedtime. As you start to pacify vata, you will help support the relaxation of the back.

Kati Basti

A wonderfully soothing and healing procedure, kati basti is used for various types of back pain and discomfort from sciatica to herniated discs. To do this, you will lie down on your belly, and a trained practitioner will make a circular flour dam on your back. Then, he will pour warm herbalized oil inside the dam. You will relax for several minutes while the warm, medicated oil sinks into your skin and into the body.

For Acne

Acne can be the result of emotional, hormonal, or bacterial causes. It's important to find out what the cause is so it can be properly treated. By all accounts, whatever the root cause, it signifies aggravated pitta. Pitta moves under the skin and then erupts as acne (or rash, hives, eczema, etc.).

Pacify Pitta

Follow a pitta-pacifying diet. Also, don't spend time playing outside in extremely hot weather: if you want to be outside, be sure it's not during the hottest hours of the day. Practice pitta-pacifying yoga, meditation, and breathwork.

Is there an herb to take for skin breakouts?
Your Ayurvedic specialist may recommend neem. Neem is a cooling herb. Your specialist will recommend how it can be used topically on the skin and also taken internally.

Put Your Mind on Something Else

If you worry and stress about your acne, it likely will not disappear. The key is to relax and pacify pitta as often as you can in your life. So, if you start to become worried or unhappy, try to turn your attention to something that is calming and relaxing in your life. When you do think of your skin, imagine it as clear, and then take your mind off it. Take a walk outside or listen to some music that you enjoy. Learning to relax and calm the mind and body will be effective, whereas continuing to think about the acne will aggravate it.

For Insomnia

There are a number of remedies you can try to help with trouble falling asleep and staying asleep. One thing to start doing is to avoid stimluating activites starting at least one hour before bed. That means no television, no computer, and no overly stimulating reading material. Do relaxing activities, such as listening to soothing music, reading books that aren't disturbing, or listening to a yoga nidra CD. You can take a warm bath, do a self-massage, or sit outside and look at the stars.

Soothing Drinks

Make yourself a cup of warm milk. Add spice to it, such as a teaspoon of turmeric, a teaspoon of nutmeg, and a teaspoon of cinnamon. Add ½ tablespoon of ghee, and you've got yourself a soothing bedtime drink.

If you don't like milk, you can also enjoy a cup of chamomile tea or peppermint tea before bed.

ESSENTIAL

When you prepare yourself a calming drink before bed, keep your attention on enjoying the beverage and noticing the quiet of nighttime. Allow yourself to sink into the peacefulness of the night and the warmth of the drink. Slowly take sips, and notice how it makes you feel. Don't watch television or do stimulating activities: that counteracts the effect.

Oil the Feet

A self-massage before bed is a relaxing way to transition from an active mind to a body ready for rest. It's especially effective to massage your feet with oil, slowly, rhythmically, and with mindfulness. Take your time as you rub oil into the soles and heels of your feet. Pay special attention to the toes. Wind down with this nourishing bedtime ritual.

For Nosebleeds

According to Dr. Lad, nosebleeds are considered pitta. To balance the heat, use cooling remedies to effectively stop a nosebleed. There can be many causes, and as with all symptoms, if some simple remedies do not help, you must see a doctor. While many nosebleeds can be simple to stop because they are from dryness in the nasal passages, allergies, or stress, some nosebleeds can be caused by more serious conditions. If after trying several remedies the nosebleed doesn't stop, see a doctor.

If You Have a Nosebleed, Relax

One of the most important things you can do, especially while doing these recommended rememdies, is relax. Nosebleeds can be aggravated by stress. Stand or sit up (lying down can cause more bleeding), and relax. Breathe deep into the belly to help encourage the relaxation response. Relax.

Use Cold Water

To stop a nosebleed, it will help to cool the nose and cool yourself internally to balance pitta. Try these methods.

1. Drink a glass of cool water.
2. Rinse a clean washcloth in cool water, and use it as a compress for the forehead and nose.
3. Very gently blow the nose to get out any obstruction that may be causing the nosebleed, then place a cube of ice (wrapped in a towel) on the side of the nose that is bleeding.

Each of these options is very cooling, so even just doing one will usually stop a nosebleed.

Other Remedies to Try

If cooling the nose and body isn't enough to stop the nosebleed, pinch the nose for a few moments. Don't tilt your head back, just pinch the nose. Usually after three to five minutes the bleeding will stop.

ESSENTIAL

Ghee to the rescue again! Ghee is hemostatic; it stops bleeding. Warm up some ghee and put a few drops into the nose if other methods aren't working. You can also put some ghee on a cotton swab and carefully swab inside the nostrils. Be gentle; you don't need to cause more irritation in the nose.

Pomegranate and cranberry juices can also stop nosebleeds. You can both drink the juice and put a few drops into the nose to stop bleeding.

Prevent Nosebleeds—Keep the Nose Moist

After you've stopped the nosebleed, do you what you can to prevent nosebleeds by keeping yourself well-hydrated and making sure the rooms in your home and in your office have enough humidity (using a hot water humidifier). Also, if you use a neti pot each day or at least oil your nasal passages each day, this will help keep the nasal passages clear, clean, and lubricated.

Monitoring your stress levels will also help. Before bedtime, each night, take at least five to ten minutes to just pause and do nothing. Just sit still and consciously relax the body. To do this you can try this exercise:

FIVE-MINUTE RELAXATION BEFORE BED

1. Sit upright at the edge of the bed, or in the bed, if this is comfortable for you. If lying down is more comfortable, do so. Do not go straight to sleep.
2. As you are sitting or lying down, close your eyes. Feel the heaviness of the eyelids; notice how closing the eyes helps you shut out the distractions of the day.
3. Notice your breath, take a few deep breaths in and long exhales out. Then, return to normal breathing.
4. Gently give yourself a soothing face massage. In a slow and methodical way, rub away tension from your forehead, your temples, your jawline, and then any part of your body that needs some attention.

When you're finished, slowly slide into the bed for sleeping. Move at a slow pace; encourage a restful transition from using your senses all day. Keeping yourself relaxed and hydrated could be all you need to prevent future nosebleeds.

For Indigestion

Indigestion can be caused by many factors. So talk to your Ayurvedic specialist and determine what is causing it for you. Once you get to the root of the indigestion, you will be able to prevent it. You and your specialist will be able to determine if you are experiencing vata, pitta, or kapha indigestion. Talking with her and dealing with the doshic imbalance will have long-term effects, which is better than dealing with indigestion only when it happens.

Helping Digestion with Ginger

Once you are feeling indigestion, it is likely caused by low digestive fire. Drinking a cup of ginger tea a half hour before meals is a great way to stoke the digestive fire. If you initiate your digestive fire this way before eating, you help your body prepare to digest food.

ESSENTIAL

When you are experiencing indigestion, don't eat if you aren't hungry. Give your system some time to work out what's going on, and relax as best you can. According to Ayurveda it's always best not to eat if you aren't hungry.

Another way to take ginger is to simply chew fresh ginger. Cut a thin slice of ginger, and chew on it. Allow the taste and the juice to prepare your body for digestion.

Peppermint for Bellyache

Peppermint can be very soothing to the gut, especially if you're experiencing acidity in the digestive tract. Make peppermint tea by boiling water and pouring it over loose leaf peppermint. Allow it to steep for ten minutes. Sip slowly and become aware of the aroma and the taste of the peppermint as it goes to the site to relieve your discomfort.

Soothing the Belly with Your Healing Hands

If you are experiencing pain with indigestion, give your belly a gentle and comforting massage. Rub your belly in a clockwise motion, going up the right side of the body, across the top where the colon is, and down the left side. Repeat this for several rounds. As you do this, inhale and exhale deeply, bringing soothing energy to your digestive tract.

After doing this in the front, place your hand on your lower back—the other side of where your digestive organs reside. Send healing energy for several breaths through the backside of your body.

To Brighten Your Mood

There are many things in life that can contribute to making you feel down. Everyone's life is full of waves: times when the ride feels smooth and times when the ride feels choppy. One of the best things you can do for your overall health is to learn ways to support yourself so that you can feel a sense of calm and contentment more often, even in the midst of many waves. Of course, seek guidance from your doctors and Ayurvedic specialists so they can help you deal with your specific needs, especially if you are noticing your mood is often low and it's hard to feel content or at ease.

Food as Love and Comfort

Sometimes the phrase "comfort food" is thought of as bad for one's health. Often in the United States, "comfort food" seems to be thought of as the opposite to "healthy food." This is not necessarily true.

Instead of cutting out what you think of as comfort food, can you view more foods as comfort food? Can you begin to see anything you put into your body as meant to be comforting, nourishing, and worth smiling about? There's nothing wrong with eating and feeling comforted by the food you eat, when you eat well. Eating can boost your mood and make you feel better. Eating well makes it easier for you to see life clearly, be in the present moment, and think of ways to deal with life's challenges. According to Ayurveda, when you eat right for your type and in the right amount, food is medicine. It gives you mental and physical energy, and this will help stabilize mood swings. Even when you eat foods that cause imbalance, enjoy that food, too, as you eat it. It will make it easier to digest food well when you enjoy eating.

The healthy way to begin to see food as comfort is to find out what is right for your body, by talking to your doctors and your Ayurvedic specialist. Learn what you need to do to change eating habits if necessary. For example, you could be addicted to sugar, so you may have to cut back on that for a while. In the short run, you might miss the sugar because of its quick highs, but very soon you will get used to receiving your energy in a healthier, longer-lasting way. Sugar highs are short-lived and lead to a host of health problems. Natural, whole foods will give you great amounts of energy, and that energy will last—you just have to try it.

Also, hydrate yourself with warm water throughout the day, and control your portion size. Then you will find that eating what you need will make you feel very well. If you have been eating poorly for a while, it might take some time to get your body on track, and once you do, you will be able to brighten your mood by eating well. This supports your health and mood in the short and long run.

Feel Balanced, Graceful, and at Ease

Sometimes a mood brightener doesn't have to be something stimulating. Shifting your energy from a bit gloomy or a little frustrated can be as simple as a calming yoga posture known as Crane Pose. When you practice this pose, you increase your focus, strength, balance, grace, and lightness. You also get blood moving in the body, which will really help your mood if you've been sitting for a while.

CRANE POSE

1. Come into standing, and hold on to the back of a chair if you need to for balance.
2. Feel your feet rooting into the earth. Engage the leg muscles, and feel your spine elongate as you imagine the crown of your head lifting toward the ceiling.
3. Exhale, and shift your weight onto the left leg; notice how solid and sturdy that leg is.
4. Inhale, engage the abdomen muscles, and lift the right foot off the floor with the knee bent at a 90-degree angle. Keep the pelvis parallel to the ground. If you can't comfortably lift your leg 90 degrees, do not push it. Simply lift it as high as you can, not past 90 degrees. Or, rest your foot on a block or telephone books.
5. Breathe normally, and fix your gaze on a point in front of you. Keep your gaze steady and soft.

6. Bring your awareness to the strength of the left leg, the softness of your gaze, and the joy of balancing like a crane.
7. Lift your arms out to the sides, perpendicular to the body at shoulder height, with elbows and wrists slightly bent. Breathe in and out for several breaths.
8. Replace the right foot on the ground.

After doing Crane Pose, notice how you feel. Do you notice a difference in one side of the body or the other? After pausing to notice the effects of Crane Pose, do the pose on the other side.

ESSENTIAL

When you do Crane Pose, be light about it. It isn't a contest. If you can't stay balanced, it's okay. If it's not easy the first time or second time, it's okay; it will get easier. The goal is to practice coming to the pose with ease and lightness of spirit. And, with time, your balance will likely increase, and you'll be able to do the pose with more ease and lightness.

Crane Pose is something you and your children can do together. Increase the imagery when you do it. Talk about seeing the water around you, the colors of the sunrise in front you, etc.

Move That Body!

If a more stimulating shift of energy is what you need, bring more dance into your life. There are so many ways to bring dance into your life either with a guided CD or DVD, attending a class, or just listening to music and moving around the room. There isn't a right or wrong way to dance: let the music be your body's guide.

If you aren't used to dancing or letting the music inform your movement, try this. When you turn on the music, even if it's fast-paced, close your eyes and pause. Wait a few moments to let the rhythm of the beat and the sounds affect your body; you don't have to think about it. And, then, after several moments, allow yourself to move in any way you like. The body knows what it needs; it will inform you. Again, do it with a light attitude—there's no one judging you. Smile as your body flows through space, and allow your mood to shift.

Get Moving with Your Children

Children can use the above tips just as adults can. Include your children in health-affirming exercises; this teaches them habits that they will have for their entire lives. For example, when you need to wind down before bed, include your children—teach them to wind down, too. Model the behavior to them, even at times when they don't want to or won't cooperate. When you prioritize winding down, they will notice. Even if they don't respond right away, your actions will make an impression.

The same goes for doing yoga poses to take a pause in your day or dancing around the room for stress relief and playfulness. Taking breaks is not a frivolous practice. There is time for focus, and there is time for play. The mind and body need breaks for restoration and proper functioning. Let your children see you and join you in creating that sense of balance in life.

Other Remedies from Your Specialist

Ayurveda has natural remedies for many other common and chronic conditions, from tummy aches to headaches, menstrual cramps to prostate concerns. Whatever you are going through, you can talk to your specialist about. Although you can use natural foods and herbs to support your healing process, it's best to do this under the guidance of a trained professional. You can work together to determine the underlying causes and then decide how best to proceed in ways that will aim to pacify what needs to be pacified without aggravating something else.

Herbs Can Interact with Medication

One of the most convenient things about Ayurveda is that you will use natural herbs and foods as remedies, without side effects. It's still essential to talk to your specialist about your conditions and not try to guess what to take. Your Ayurvedic specialist will have knowledge that you may not have about how potent certain herbs are and how they interact with specific medications.

You Are Unique, and Your Remedy Will Be Unique

It's also important to talk to your specialist because each person is unique: your life, your constitution, and your diet are unique to you. In order to treat underlying causes of symptoms that show up as colds, bellyaches, muscle pain, etc., you and your specialist will talk about your current and past lifestyle and health.

ESSENTIAL

When you research vata, pitta, and kapha and learn about the elements in you, you are getting a great foundational understanding about health and wellness. You are also gaining a common language that you can use with your Ayurvedic specialist to understand your mind and body. It's important not to get overconfident with the information, however, without talking to a specialist.

Seeing a specialist will help you learn what is unique about you. Besides the qualities that you notice of how the doshas are showing up in you, there are many other factors, such as your health history and how well you are digesting your food, that your specialist will take into consideration when she determines what you can do for your health. While Ayurveda is self-empowering, it's also essential for you to talk to someone with knowledge, training, and experience in this science who can help you get into balance and really feel the benefits of perfect health.

CHAPTER 16

Activities and Healing Therapies to Create Balance

In addition to preparing and enjoying food that is balancing for you and making supportive lifestyle choices, there are more ways to support your mind, body, and energy flow. Ayurvedic bodywork, the use of gems, and chakra healing are ancient and evolving modalities to bring you into balance. What's so special about these therapies is that you can book them with a trained practitioner. So, you lie down and relax while the specialist takes care of you. (If you prefer, you can also do this healing work on yourself.)

The Importance of Creating Energetic Balance

According to Ayurveda, you need energy flowing in a balanced way through your body and mind. The proper amount of energy flow allows your brain to think clearly, your body to digest and eliminate efficiently, and your heart to feel more connected to the wisdom of the universe.

Mindfulness for Balance

Mindfulness refers to bringing your awareness to the present moment. It means paying attention to what you're doing, how you're doing it, and what's going on around you in each moment. When you're in the present moment, you can enjoy the peace of being "right here, right now," where regrets about past events or concerns about future possibilities won't cause you stress.

When your awareness is on the present moment, you can deal with what comes up more effectively, and your physical body can relax and perform its vital functions. Otherwise, when you are stressed out, your body goes into fight-or-flight mode (also called a sympathetic response): your breath becomes shallow, your heart rate increases, and many other "emergency" responses are triggered in the body. This obstructs the free and natural flow of energy in the body. So, you want to engage a parasympathetic response (also called a relaxation response). Keeping your mind at peace through mindfulness is one technique that will help.

Why Be Mindful?

When you're being mindful, you are able to enjoy, appreciate, and bene-fit from what's going on in your life in a vivid way. It means you're not primarily living in the past or in the future. Time can actually feel stretched when you live this way, and you will more thoroughly experience life. For example, when you mindfully eat—when you chew slowly, savor the tastes, and pay attention to the fact that you are eating—you will feel full after eating less than you would eat if you weren't being mindful, your body will be more powerfully affected by the experience of eating, and you'll likely remember later in the day that you've eaten.

Being mindful also means checking in with yourself to see how you are doing. When you don't check in with yourself and pay attention to your mental, emotional, and physical states, you can unknowingly start accumulating mental, emotional, and energetic debris. When you don't digest it and clear it out, then it throws you off balance. The longer you are out of balance and the more debris you hold on to, the more your overall health becomes compromised. According to Ayurveda, physical symptoms are often a result of what you experience in life and how you digest it energetically, mentally, and physically.

A Mindfulness Exercise

There are many ways to practice mindfulness. The more you practice being mindful, the more often you will start to live that way, sometimes without consciously thinking about doing it. Here's an exercise you can do as often as you like.

DAILY MINDFULNESS EXERCISE

1. When you can remember, at any point in your day, stop what you are doing for a moment.
2. With your eyes closed deepen your breath, and send your awareness to the various parts of your body starting with the top of your head and moving downward to the feet.
3. As you send awareness to each body part, inhale and imagine sending prana to that body part. Exhale, and imagine releasing stress.
4. After you've brought your awareness down to the feet, notice if anywhere in the body you feel discomfort. Make small movements of the body to release tension and stiffness.
5. Finally, take a few very deep inhalations and exhalations. On the final exhale, bring a small smile to your lips.
6. Open your eyes and take another moment to appreciate that small break.

You can take mindfulness breaks like this throughout your day; however, you don't have to take a break to practice mindfulness. You can bring mindfulness to any activity. It simply means being present with what is and being intentional about what you're doing. It might sound simple, and in fact it's surprising how often the mind isn't on what's happening right in the present moment.

Noticing Imbalance Early

When you're being mindful in your life, you're much more aware of what's going on. This means that you'll also be prone to noticing signs of imbalance early. The sooner you notice imbalance, the easier it is for you to bring yourself into a healthy state again. If imbalance persists, your physical symptoms will get worse. For example, if you ignore a cold it can turn into bronchitis or pneumonia, and the further along it goes, the more harm it does to your body. Being mindful allows you to notice what's going on with you and your environment.

Nourishing Bodywork

Bodywork is an important part of Ayurvedic healthy living. The treatments facilitate the flow of energy, blood, and lymph throughout the body. They also balance the doshas, and each has additional benefits depending on what you need. Some types of treatments and oils will stimulate energy; others will primarily calm the nervous system.

- *Abyangha* is the application of oil to your entire body. The Ayurvedic bodyworker warms oil infused with herbs, specifically selected for you. Then she applies the oil to your body in a way that supports physical and energetic circulation, loosens toxins, and relaxes the mind. It's also called Abyangha when you give yourself an Ayurvedic oil massage.
- *Abyangha-Garshana* includes a silk-glove massage before the Abyangha treatment. The silk-glove massage cleans the skin and stimulates circulation before the oil sinks in to nourish your body.
- *Vishesh* is a treatment of oil infused with herbs applied to the body in rapid, rhythmic movements. This helps facilitate energetic, arterial, and lymphatic flow throughout the body.
- *Shirodhara* is a steady stream of warm, herbalized oil poured onto the forehead, balancing and calming the mind.

Often Ayurvedic bodyworkers will combine treatments. For example, you could request Abyangha-Shirodhara.

Ayurvedic bodywork is healing for both giver and receiver. In today's stress-filled world, many people are affected by anxiety or ungroundedness, two common symptoms of excess vata. The use of warm, herbalized oil is wonderfully grounding and nurturing for vata. During an abhyanga, you are nourished from head to toe with flowing, repetitive massage strokes that calm the nervous system. It is no surprise that sneha, the word for oil in Sanskrit, also means "love." I find myself sinking into a quiet, peaceful state as I give the massage, especially if I say mantras with each stroke. After the session, the receiver is no longer restless, and will commonly have sparkling eyes and a noticeable glow in her face. She will often comment that she "has not been so relaxed in a long time," which means that the bodywork has served its purpose!
—*Sadie Cunningham, Ayurvedic massage therapist, Kripalu Center for Yoga & Health*

To find a trained practitioner near you, look for Ayurvedic specialists in your area who can do the bodywork or who can recommend where to have it done. Also, some spas and retreat centers are now offering Ayurvedic treatments, chakra balancing, and other therapies that balance your energy and support the body.

Understanding the Chakras

Chakra simply means "wheel" or "disc," and the seven major chakras in your body are spinning energy wheels where energy pathways converge. You have other chakras in the body and beyond the body in your energy field. The ancient rishis discovered that by meditating on the seven major chakras in ascending order, they could awaken and move kundalini energy through their physical and energetic bodies. It was through this type of meditation that they would reach liberation or enlightenment.

Chakra Theory's Evolution

One thing that chakra theory has in common with Ayurveda is that it evolves as times change. One of the important attributes of Ayurveda is that as it embraces new knowledge it retains its ancient wisdom. Ayurveda has always been about observing what's happening in the natural world and how human beings are a part of the natural order, and as important new discoveries come about, Ayurveda adapts and remains authentic and deeply rooted in ancient wisdom. For example, an Ayurvedic doctor may be trained in both Western medicine and Ayurveda so that she can use them as complementary.

FACT

The secrets of chakra meditation were passed on orally for an unknown number of years before they were put into writing. The first known written account of chakra theory is in Sanskrit, from the year 1577. In 1919, Sir John Woodroffe (pen name, Arthur Avalon) was the first to publish an English translation of that Sanskrit text, in *Serpent Power*.

Chakra theory is also an ancient body of knowledge that grows with more research, contemplation, and observation. Chakra theory has expanded significantly in the past few centuries, revealing more about how the chakras tie in to specific psychological and biological processes.

How Balancing Chakras Balances You

Beginning thousands of years ago, rishis and their students meditated on the seven chakras as a path to clearing karma and reaching enlightenment. Chakra theory came to the West in the early twentieth century, and soon after, the first translation of chakra theory was available. Theosophists took great interest. They began experimenting and discovering how the chakras are connected to biological processes. Their discoveries further illuminate the connection between how freely energy flows in the body and how healthy and youthful a person is.

ESSENTIAL

In the twentieth century, interest in how the chakras affect a person's psychology has been expounded greatly and with great erudition by Anodea Judith, who has written books and produced a beautifully animated DVD on the chakras.

When the chakras are balanced, it means that energy is flowing in the body in a way that is neither too fast nor too slow. It means that you are firing on all cylinders. Your mind and body are being fed with just the right amount of life-force energy, or prana, to keep you functioning with optimum clarity, ease, contentment, and focus.

When any of the chakras is out of balance, it's spinning too sluggishly or too quickly. What affects the chakras' ability to function are the same factors that affect your overall health: your lifestyle, your emotional and mental state, and how you're treating your physical body through diet, movement, and stress management. Your health has a symbiotic relationship with the health of the chakras. If you are feeling unbalanced it can throw them off balance, and if they are out of balance it will cause you to be off balance.

Chakras and the Elements

The chakras each have a stem in the spine, and they flower out into the body. In the following table, you will see the name of each chakra, its general placement that you can use for beginning visualizations, and the element that it's linked to.

▼ CHAKRAS AND THE ELEMENTS

Chakra	Placement	Element
Root	perineum	earth
Svadhistana	sacrum	water
Manipura	solar plexus	fire
Anahata	heart	air
Visuddha	throat	ether
Ajna	third eye	mind
Sahasrara	crown of the head	consciousness

Identifying chakras in this way with the elements, you can get a sense of how they are connected to the doshas.

Chakras and the Doshas

Use the elements as the unifying factor between the chakras and the doshas to help you understand how to use chakra healing to balance the doshas.

For example, if you're feeling ungrounded that is a sign of vata imbalance. So, you want to bring energy to the chakras that will help you feel grounded. The first chakra is of the earth element; it is grounding. The second chakra is of water, which is also balancing for vata. The third chakra is fire, heating. So, if you're feeling excess vata, you need to bring more energy to those lower chakras to help you feel grounded.

QUOTE

Ayurvedic psychology balances Vata, Pitta, and Kapha in the body and increases Sattva in the mind to harmonize lower chakra functions and create the foundation for the opening of their higher potential. Tejas helps open the lower chakras and corresponds to Kundalini. Ojas aids in the unfoldment of the higher chakras of the head and third eye. Prana allows the heart (air) chakra to open. —Dr. David Frawley, *Ayurveda and the Mind*

Pitta can be related to the solar plexus chakra and third eye (fire, intellect, and connection to wisdom). With pitta as predominant, you may feel disconnected from the subtle, profound energies associated with the heart and throat chakras. When it comes to these chakras, you will be a good public speaker and advocate, but perhaps you will have trouble with true connection and good, comfortable communication in personal and intimate relationships.

Kapha energy can be linked to the root and sacral chakras. If you're predominantly kapha, you may not have a strong manipura chakra, which will affect your digestive fire as well as your self-esteem. Bring some of that energy up from the root and sacral chakras to energize the manipura and higher chakras.

Simple Chakra Healing Exercise

There are several resources available to learn various simple, engaging, and practical chakra healing methods that you can do in your own home, with your children, or by yourself. Here is one simple method for bringing energy to the various chakras.

Visualizing the color associated with each chakra is one way to energize that chakra. The colors typically affect chakras with this pairing.

- Root chakra and the color red
- Sacral chakra and the color orange
- Solar plexus chakra and the color yellow
- Heart chakra and the color green
- Throat chakra and the color blue
- Third eye chakra and the color indigo
- Crown chakra and the colors white, purple, or gold

The order of these colors corresponds to the colors of the visible rainbow from bottom to top. When you would like to bring energy to a particular chakra, envision the corresponding color glowing brightly in the area of that chakra. Try this visualization:

1. Sit with your sitting bones rooted into the chair or earth.
2. Elongate the spine so you are sitting up straight and the crown of your head is pointing toward the ceiling.
3. Relax the jaw, relax the arms, relax the belly.
4. Deepen your inhalations and exhalations.
5. On an inhale envision drawing the color red in through your nostrils and way down deep into the perineum.
6. On the exhale, exhale slowly, imagining any muddy color leaving the body.
7. Repeat this two more times, envisioning the color red going into the region of the perineum.
8. Do this visualization at each chakra, with its corresponding color. Inhale that color deep into the appropriate area, and exhale any unwanted energy.
9. When you get to the crown chakra, on your final exhale, return to normal breathing.
10. Breathe normally for a few moments, noticing the effects of the visualization. Then, open your eyes.

This is a visualization you can do for all the chakras. Even if it seems that just one chakra is out of balance, it is always helpful to give attention to each chakra because all chakras do affect each other.

FACT

This is a great activity to do with children, in partners. Have your child lie on the ground, faceup or facedown. Hold your hand a few inches away from the child's body and visualize sending red energy into the root chakra. Then, move your hand up to where the sacral chakra is located, and visualize sending orange light. Continue this up the body, and tell the child to envision the colors entering her body at each location so she can participate.

There are so many ways to support your chakras, and learning from someone who has been trained and practices chakra healing can help you along your chakra healing journey. Also, a trained healer will be able to notice things about your chakras that you may not be able to notice until you have more practice. See Appendix B for additional resources on healing the chakras.

Using Gems for Healing

Ayurvedic wisdom teaches about healing properties in gems. The following are general guidelines about gems. In general, it's important for you to talk to someone who is well-trained in this aspect of Ayurveda for the most effective advice about what would be most supportive to you. When you talk to a specialist, he can help make sure you choose the right gems, that you wear them on the appropriate finger (or as a necklace), and that you choose an appropriate setting.

The Healing Power of Gems

Like all things of nature, gems carry energy. Gem therapy is energetic therapy—energy from the gem interacts with your energy field. Gems help support you with energy that you need where you are deficient.

Many gems will absorb the energy around them, so it's important to cleanse your gems before you use them or wear them. After they are cleansed, they are restored with their own healing energy, and any other energy they may have picked up has been washed away.

To cleanse a gem that is not water-soluble, find a spring or another type of natural water source. Bring your gem to the natural water source, and rinse it under the fresh water for a few moments. Pull the gem out of the water, and state your healing intentions.

Each gem has energy that heals a particular aspect of you. See the following table, showing how Ayurveda categorizes the gems.

▼ **GEMS AND THEIR HEALING POWER**

Gem	Uses
Diamond	imagination, love
Emerald	perception, discernment
Pearl	mental calm, serenity
Red Coral	vitality
Ruby	self-esteem
Sapphire (blue)	independence, patience
Sapphire (yellow)	wisdom, creativity

For less expensive versions of the above gems try:

- Clear quartz for diamond
- Jade for emerald
- Moonstone for pearl
- Garnet for ruby
- Lapis lazuli for blue sapphire
- Citrine for yellow sapphire

There are other gems, too, with additional healing properties. For as many conditions as the human body can exhibit, there are gems to help. Your specialist in vedic astrology, **jyotish**, will be able to guide you.

Gems and Astrology

Because the planet Earth is in relationship with other planets and influenced by these energetic relationships, so is each person. Therefore, it may come as no surprise that there is a branch of astrology in Ayurveda.

According to vedic astrology, you would wear the gems that you need to create balance and harmony within you according to your energetic relationship to the energy of the configuration of the planets.

Gems can also be used because of how they affect doshas in you. Based on the energies of the planets, certain gems will balance or aggravate certain doshas. For example, blue sapphire calms vata and kapha, and opal calms pitta.

Aside from wearing gems, you can also make water infused with their healing energy. To do this, place a flawless gem in clear, spring water overnight. The next day, sip the water to receive the benefits. The water will be energized with the healing qualities of that gem. This is a great way to receive energy from gems, in the meantime, before talking to a specialist for more specific advice that is personalized for you.

Marma Therapy

Marmas are sensitive energetic zones in and on the body. Marma means "vulnerable" or "sensitive." You can use marma therapy to facilitate the flow of prana or to stop the flow of prana at particular sites on the body. In other words, you can focus on marma points to heal a person's ailments, and you could use them to end a person's life. The marma points are taught to students of martial arts (for self-defense), and they are taught to students of Ayurveda and yoga as powerful sites that can set in motion deep healing.

Where Are Marmas?

The major Ayurvedic texts list 51 marma regions and 107 marma points. (The number of points is greater than the number of regions because some regions have more than one point, and also to reach some regions there is a point on the back of the body and the front of the body.) Marmas cover the entire body, and many Ayurvedic teachers recognize more than 107 marma points.

Are marma points the same as acupuncture points?
Marma points are like acupuncture points in that they both are places where you can facilitate deep healing. However, they don't correlate exactly in location or in number. Also, marmas can be larger than acupuncture points, and the therapies move energy in a different way—in Ayurveda marmas are usually worked on during bodywork/massage sessions, not with needles.

The ancient texts list specific places where you can find marmas throughout the body, but remember that Ayurveda acknowledges everyone as an individual. The exact location of marmas will be different (at least slightly) for each person. When sending healing energy to the body, the prana will find its way into the places where prana is very low. Just as water flows where there is space, prana flows to where it's needed. The points listed in the textbooks are useful as a guide, a point of departure and understanding. The interaction between the healer and the patient will reveal where the most sensitive spots are for that person.

Marmas and the Doshas

Marma therapy can be used for all doshas and can treat a variety of imbalances that are associated with particular doshas. For vata dosha, marma therapy can have many balancing effects, including:

❑ Relieving pain in bones and joints
❑ Calming anxiety
❑ Promoting sleep
❑ Relieving constipation

For pitta dosha, again, there are many benefits, which include:

❑ Calming anger
❑ Reducing acidity in the small intestine
❑ Cleansing the blood

Marma therapy can relieve kapha symptoms, including:

❑ Increasing mental and physical energy
❑ Clearing mucus
❑ Stimulating weight loss

All Ayurvedic therapies benefit from the knowledge of marma therapy because it works directly with prana in the body. Using the marma points correctly, you can increase or decrease heat in the body, as well as address long-term and degenerative disease.

You can also use knowledge of marma points to understand your own energy body. It can help you in your yoga practice and with your self-massage. One thorough guide for learning the placement of the marmas and how to work with them is *Ayurveda and Marma Therapy* by Dr. David Frawley, Dr. Subhash Ranade, and Dr. Avinash Lele.

Mudras

Another very effective and creative way to move energy through the body is to use hand mudras, or postures for the hands. This can also be practiced with children because it's fun to hold the hands in different positions and envision the energy flowing through the body.

FACT

You don't have to be sitting to use mudras. You can stand, walk, or even dance while you hold your hands in specific postures. Bringing joy and creativity to energetic healing makes it a special addition to your day rather than something you feel you have to do.

Each mudra is used for a particular purpose. The way you hold your hands activates different marmas and also directs energy to different parts of the body.

Hand Mudra for Inner Harmony

In her book *Mudras: Yoga in your Hands*, Gertrud Hirschi explains how to do a variety of mudras. This posture, Matangi, is for inner harmony and rulership.

MATANGI MUDRA

1. Bring the palms of the hands together.
2. With fingers and palms touching, spread the fingers.
3. Fold the fingers of the right and left hand all the way down so you interlace the fingers.
4. With the fingers of the hands interlaced and folded down, extend the two middle fingers up, and allow them to press against each other.
5. Hold for several breaths, then release the posture.

According to Hirschi, you should do this posture as needed or three times per day for four minutes. This mudra brings balance to the solar plexus, to the heart, and to the process of digestion. All of these benefits enhance your Ayurvedic lifestyle.

In addition, this mudra stimulates the earth element, which is an element of kapha. So, it will help ground vata and pitta and bring some extra support to kapha. All of the doshas can use the pranic support that this mudra sends to the regions of the body and to the process of digestion.

Hand Mudra to Help Energy Flow in Joints

Joint pain is often called "chronic" and can especially affect those with vata imbalance. Having a mudra that you can practice is an easy option to help energy flow. You do have to be diligent with it. Hirschi recommends holding this posture four times a day for fifteen minutes each time. She also recommends that if there is illness, you should hold the mudra twice as long, six times per day.

MUDRA TO RELIEVE JOINT PAIN

1. Open the right hand, and touch the thumb to the ring finger.
2. Open the left hand and touch the thumb to the middle finger.
3. Hold both hands like this, and breathe normally. Envision and enjoy the healing flow of energy.

Mudras, like other yoga poses and other forms of energetic healing, may take some time to work. Sometimes you'll feel immediate relief, other times you may not. Some of the benefits of doing mudras (rather than taking over-the-counter or prescription drugs) is that mudras are all natural, there are no side effects, you will not become physically dependent on them, and they are free!

CHAPTER 17

Recipes for Breakfast

Pumpkin Pancakes

This recipe is good for balancing vata and pitta, and it will increase kapha.

INGREDIENTS | SERVES 4

1½ cups organic milk

2 eggs

1 (15-ounce) can organic pumpkin puree

4 tablespoons vegetable oil

½ cup maple syrup

2 cups all-purpose flour

2 teaspoons baking powder

1 teaspoon baking soda

Mixture of: 1 teaspoon ground cinnamon, 1 teaspoon ground nutmeg, 1 teaspoon ground ginger, ¼ teaspoon ground clove

½ teaspoon salt

4 tablespoons organic butter

1. In a large mixing bowl, beat milk and eggs together well.

2. Add pumpkin puree, oil, and maple syrup.

3. In a separate bowl, combine all the dry ingredients.

4. Stir into the pumpkin mixture. If it's too thick, add a little bit of milk at a time, until it becomes the desired consistency.

5. Melt 1 tablespoon of butter on a large cast-iron skillet until it starts to smoke.

6. Pour about ½ cup batter for each pancake onto the skillet.

7. Cook over medium heat until bubbles form on top of the pancake, then flip the pancake and brown it on the other side.

8. Keep pancakes to the side and warm while you cook the other pancakes.

9. Before serving, top with butter and maple syrup. (You can also dust them with powdered sugar and/or cinnamon.)

Summer Vegetable Frittata

You can add any vegetables you'd like to for this frittata. It's best to choose the vegetables that are in season.

INGREDIENTS | SERVES 4

3 cloves garlic, minced

1 leek cleaned well, diced

2 tablespoons olive oil

1 teaspoon Italian seasoning mix

1 teaspoon crushed rosemary leaves

1 pound of a mixture of fresh broccoli, cauliflower, zucchini, spinach, yellow and red peppers

4 large organic eggs

1 cup grated cheese (whatever your preference, such as Swiss or Cheddar)

2 tablespoons grated Parmesan cheese

Salt and pepper, to taste

Making Changes Depending on Your Consitution

For vata, use ghee instead of olive oil for sautéing the vegetables, and be sure to really cook the vegetables well. Also, pick your cheese based on your dosha. Most dairy is good for vata, soft cheeses are best for pitta, and kaphas could do all right with goat's cheese. Goat's cheese would be a great choice if you're serving to people with a variety of constitutions.

1. In a 10-inch heavy skillet, sauté garlic and leeks in olive oil over medium heat until they start to brown.

2. Add the seasonings and vegetables. Sauté until tender, about 5 minutes.

3. Whisk the eggs with a tablespoon of cold water until the yolks and whites are combined.

4. Pour egg mixture evenly over vegetables in the skillet.

5. Sprinkle cheeses evenly over the top.

6. Reduce heat to low. Cover and continue cooking until eggs are set, approximately 3 to 5 minutes.

7. Cut into wedges, and serve. Add salt and pepper, to taste.

Kitchari

Kitchari is a traditional Ayurvedic dish that can be made in a very basic way (such as this recipe demonstrates). You can also add vegetables to the dish, choosing vegetables that will bring balance to your constitution.

INGREDIENTS | SERVES 4–6

4 tablespoons ghee

3 teaspoons each of turmeric, cumin, and coriander

5 cups water

1 cup basmati rice

1 cup mung dahl

2 bay leaves

Salt and pepper, to taste

Kitchari Is Easy to Digest

Kitchari is very easy on the digestive system. It's well-cooked and full of grains, protein, and anti-inflammatory spices. It's a perfect meal to eat if you want to give your system a rest. There are many variations of kitchari, and a version is used as the main sustenance for someone doing panchakarma—the extended, supervised process of detoxifying the body at its deepest levels.

1. Rinse mung dahl and rice.

2. In a large pot, melt the ghee and add turmeric, cumin, and coriander. Stir for 2 minutes until fragrant.

3. Stir in mung dahl and mix very well.

4. Carefully pour 5 cups of water over the mixture and bring to a boil.

5. Take the heat down to a simmer, and simmer lightly covered for a half hour.

6. Add the rice, bay leaves, and add more boiling water if necessary. Cook the entire mixture until the rice is done, about another half hour.

7. When the rice is soft, the kitchari is done. Serve, and add extra ghee for calming vata and/or salt and pepper, to taste.

Cacao Morning Bliss

*This cacao drink is great for breakfast or any time of day for a snack.
Notice, too, there's no refined sugar, no gluten, and no dairy.*

INGREDIENTS | SERVES 2

2 cups fresh spring water

1½ tablespoons cacao (not cocoa) powder

1 banana

Handful of fresh blueberries

1 teaspoon honey

½ teaspoon cinnamon

1. Blend all ingredients together in a blender.

2. Pour into 2 glasses, and enjoy.

Cacao's Fortifying Properties

Hernan Cortes conquered what is now Mexico City in 1521, and the previous ruler was a confirmed lover of chocolate. Cortes himself wrote, "The divine drink which builds up resistance and fights fatigue. A cup of this precious drink permits a man to walk for a whole day without food."

CHAPTER 18

Main Courses
for Lunch and Dinner

Soba Noodles and Sun-Dried Tomatoes

If you buy sun-dried tomatoes that are dehydrated, rehydrate them for this recipe. To do this, pour boiling water over them, cover, and let them sit for 5 to 10 minutes.

INGREDIENTS | SERVES 4

1 (8-ounce) pack of soba noodles

1 onion, chopped

2 tablespoons olive oil

3 cloves garlic, minced

10 sun-dried tomatoes, sliced

½ cup of black olives, chopped

½ bunch of kale, rinsed

½ bunch of chard, rinsed

2 cups fresh spinach, rinsed

Olive oil, goat cheese, salt, and pepper, to taste

Great Dish for All Doshas

Soba noodles are great for kapha because they are 100 percent buckwheat, which is hot, light, and dry. Generally, vatas wouldn't do well with these noodles, but this recipe has other ingredients to balance vata, including olive oil, garlic, black olives, and goat cheese. Pittas will do well with the balance for them that includes kale, olives, onion, and olive oil.

1. Boil enough water to cook soba noodles and pour over sun-dried tomatoes if they need to be rehydrated.

2. Cook the soba noodles as directed on the package.

3. While noodles are cooking, sauté onions in the olive oil until the onions are transluscent.

4. To the onions, add garlic, sun-dried tomatoes, and black olives. Sauté for 5 minutes.

5. Add kale, chard, and spinach to the other vegetables. Cover and steam until the greens are wilted. Uncover and remove from heat.

6. Once noodles are done, strain; then mix all the cooked ingredients together.

7. Toss with olive oil, goat cheese, salt, and pepper, to taste.

Lunch Burrito

Instead of using brown rice in this recipe, you can use any grain of your choice. Try quinoa or white rice for variations. You can also choose to add beans or tofu for a legume or chicken if you'd like meat. Instead of broccoli, you can substitute kale or chard.

INGREDIENTS | SERVES 2

2 whole wheat or rice tortillas

Your dressing of choice (balsamic vinegar dressing, mustard, or spicy peanut sauce)

2 cups cooked brown rice

1 cup broccoli cut into bite-sized pieces

2 medium carrots, shredded

½ cucumber, chopped

1½ cups bean sprouts

1 cup toasted walnuts

Goat cheese, optional

Salt and pepper, to taste

1. Warm tortillas in the oven or toaster oven for a few moments until they are soft.

2. Lay each tortilla flat on a plate. Spread dressing on the tortilla.

3. Wrap the rice, vegetables, walnuts, and goat cheese in the tortilla. Salt and pepper, to taste.

Make It Vata Pacifying

To make it even better for vata, cook the ingredients (except the cucumber) before putting them in the burrito, and see what you think of coating the tortilla with ghee or a grounding dressing before adding the filling.

Gourmet Squash

You can garnish the top of the squash with the squash seeds. Roast the seeds in olive oil on a separate baking dish while the squash is baking, and as the final step, sprinkle the seeds on top.

Turn This Into a Dessert

This recipe is a nourishing meal. For a sweet and simple variation, as in dessert, change it up. After you remove the seeds from the squash and coat the insides of the squash with ghee, sprinkle cinnamon on the squash. Bake the squash the same way, and when you take it out, you'll have a sweet dessert. Drizzle honey on it, too, to pacify vata in the cold winter months.

1. Preheat the oven to 375°F.

2. Remove the seeds from the acorn squash, and put the seeds aside. Coat the inside of the squash halves with ghee or butter. Place the squash halves faceup in the baking pan in about ½ inch of water. Cook until the squash is soft and the edges are brown. This will take about 45 minutes.

3. While the squash is baking, sauté the kale in ghee or olive oil until it's wilted. Add rice and cranberries and continue to sauté for 2 minutes.

4. Stuff squash with the rice mixture, add some goat cheese on top, and bake for another 10 minutes.

Indian Chickpeas

This can be served over your favorite grain, with greens, or as filling for a lunch burrito.

INGREDIENTS | SERVES 2

2 tablespoons ghee, olive oil, or butter

1 medium onion, chopped

3 cloves garlic (optional)

1 teaspoon of each: cumin, coriander, and cardamom

1 tablespoon cumin seeds

2 cups chickpeas

3 fresh tomatoes or 1 (14.5-ounce) can tomatoes, diced

Salt, to taste

1. Place the ghee, olive oil, or butter in a large skillet over medium heat, add onions, and sauté until they are translucent. Add garlic and spices and continue to sauté for 3 minutes.

2. Add chickpeas and tomatoes. Stir, and let simmer for 15 to 20 minutes.

3. Add salt to taste.

Simply Baked Salmon

Salmon is particularly good for vata types. Tamari helps balance vata and pitta, but it's not the best for kapha. The garlic, lime, and scallion will be beneficial for kapha.

INGREDIENTS | SERVES 2–4

⅔ cup tamari

2 teaspoons toasted sesame oil

2 tablespoons grated ginger

Juice of 1 lime

4 garlic cloves, minced

4 scallions, finely chopped

2–3 pounds freshwater Alaskan sockeye salmon filet

¼ cup water

1. Combine tamari, sesame oil, ginger, lime, garlic, and scallions in a bowl to make a marinade.

2. Place the salmon in a shallow baking dish, and pour the marinade over it. Refrigerate for 2–3 hours.

3. Preheat oven to 375°F.

4. Place salmon in covered glass baking dish. Add water so fish can steam.

5. Place the salmon in the oven and bake to your liking, about 20–25 minutes or until just opaque in the center (the salmon will continue to cook when you remove it from the oven).

Wild Rice Pecan Pilaf

This dish can be served on its own as a main course with vegetables on the side, or it can be served as a side dish to a main course (such as the Simply Baked Salmon).

INGREDIENTS | SERVES 4

1½ cups brown basmati rice

½ cup wild rice

4 cups water

2 tablespoons ghee or olive oil

1 clove garlic, minced

1 medium carrot, diced

2 stalks of celery, diced

3–5 scallions, diced

1 teaspoon fresh rosemary

1 teaspoon fresh thyme

Salt and pepper, to taste

⅓ cup roasted pecans

1. Rinse rice. Cover rice with water in a 1:2 ratio. Add 1 tablespoon ghee or olive oil. Bring the rice to a boil; then cover and simmer until the rice is done, approximately 35 minutes. Check on the rice occasionally to make sure there is enough water; do not stir.

2. While rice is cooking, sauté the garlic, carrots, and celery for 5 minutes in the remaining tablespoon of ghee or olive oil. Then add the scallions, rosemary, and thyme. Sauté for 3 to 5 more minutes.

3. Add this mixture to the rice after the rice is cooked.

4. Add salt and pepper, to taste.

5. Add roasted pecans, and serve.

Asparagus Risotto

Instead of using organic butter for this recipe, you can use ghee.

INGREDIENTS | SERVES 2 AS A MAIN COURSE, 4 AS A SIDE DISH

1 pound thin asparagus

4 tablespoons organic butter

4 large garlic cloves, minced

1 medium-sized leek, cleaned and chopped fine

1 cup Arborio rice, rinsed

3½ cups organic chicken broth

1 tablespoon lemon juice

½ cup freshly grated Parmesan cheese

Salt and pepper, to taste

1. Break off and discard any tough ends from asparagus. Cut asparagus into thirds.

2. Blanch asparagus in boiling water for 3 minutes, then run under cold water to stop cooking. Drain.

3. Melt 3 tablespoons butter in heavy saucepan. Add garlic and leeks, cooking until translucent.

4. Add rice and cook over medium heat, stirring continuously until kernels glisten and are coated with butter.

5. Add chicken broth, about ½ cup at a time. Stir constantly, adding more liquid when the previous ½ cup is absorbed. This should take about 20 minutes. Rice should be a little firm but still tender.

6. Add lemon juice and asparagus. Stir and cook another 2 minutes.

7. Remove from heat. Stir in remaining butter and Parmesan cheese. Add salt and pepper, to taste.

Hijiki, with Tofu, Carrots, and Onions

Hijiki, when rinsed like this, decreases vata and has a neutral effect on pitta and kapha.

INGREDIENTS | SERVES 4–6

¾ cup dried hijiki

½ pound block of medium or hard tofu

4 tablespoons sesame oil

1 carrot, quartered lengthwise then cut into quartered rounds

1 onion, diced

2 cups vegetable broth

3 tablespoons tamari

What's So Great about Hijiki?

Hijiki won't aggravate any of the doshas, and it's a good source of calcium, iron, and magnesium. It's a sea vegetable that goes well when paired with land vegetables, especially carrots.

1. Soak hijiki in a large bowl of water for about an hour. It will swell to about 5 times its original volume. Drain well; rinse until water runs clean. Set aside.

2. Cut tofu into 1-inch slices and fry in 3 tablespoons sesame oil until lightly browned on both sides. Cube. Set aside.

3. Sauté carrots and onion in remaining tablespoon of sesame oil until soft.

4. Add well-drained hijiki and tofu to carrot and onion mixture.

5. Add broth and tamari. Bring to a boil. Simmer over low heat until hijiki is tender—about 20 to 30 minutes, adding a little water if needed.

6. Serve as a side dish or main course.

Pesto Pizza on Sprouted Tortilla

This recipe can be used as a meal or as a snack because the crust is thin and light. To turn it into a more substantial meal, add more toppings, such as more vegetables, chicken, or cheese.

INGREDIENTS | SERVES 2

2 cups fresh basil, lightly packed
3 medium cloves garlic
¼ cup extra-virgin olive oil
⅓ cup walnuts
½ cup freshly grated Parmesan cheese
2 Ezekiel brand sprouted tortillas
2 cups fresh spinach

1. Preheat oven or toaster oven to 400°F.

2. Rinse basil and peel garlic.

3. Chop garlic in a food processor with some of the olive oil.

4. Add walnuts and some more of the olive oil to the food processor; blend.

5. Add the basil and more of the olive oil; blend.

6. Add the Parmesan cheese and more olive oil; blend.

7. Slowly keep adding olive oil and blending until basil is a smooth paste. Set aside.

8. Brush both sides of a tortilla with olive oil. Place tortilla on lightly greased baking sheet.

9. Spread a layer of the pesto on the tortilla. Rinse the spinach and tear it into bite-sized pieces. Toss the spinach in olive oil, and place it on top of the pizza.

10. Bake in oven for 5 minutes or until the edges are golden brown and curled up.

11. Remove the pizza from the oven, and allow it to cool for a few moments.

Side Dishes and Sauces

Root Veggie Bake

You can vary the spices for this recipe. For example, you can try an Italian twist, an Indian twist, or just use salt and pepper. Even with just salt and pepper, these vegetables have their own delicious flavors.

INGREDIENTS | SERVES 4

1 large parsnip
3 medium carrots
8 small red potatotes
2 yams
1 medium onion
8 cloves of garlic, peeled
Olive oil, to lightly coat vegetables
Fresh rosemary, chopped
Salt and pepper, to taste

Tailor It to Your Constitution

To make this heavy and oily for vata, add a helping of ghee to the vegetables after they are baked. Be sure to add pepper to help stimulate digestion for vata and kapha types. For pitta, in particular, go easy on the salt and garlic. Since the garlic will be in whole cloves, a pitta type can avoid them all together.

1. Preheat the oven to 375°F.

2. Cut the vegetables into bite-sized pieces; leave the garlic cloves whole.

3. Place all the vegetables into a bowl, drizzle them with olive oil, add fresh rosemary, and gently mix until the vegetables are coated with oil.

4. Place the vegetables in baking dish, cover, and bake in the oven for about 45 minutes.

5. Stir the vegetables periodically to prevent sticking and to make sure they are cooked on all sides.

6. When the onions are brown and the other vegetables are soft, remove from oven. Add salt and pepper, to taste.

Hummus

This is a fast and easy recipe, and hummus can be used as a side dish or inside a lunch burrito. It's great to serve as an appetizer or afternoon snack, too.

INGREDIENTS | SERVES 4

2 cups dried chickpeas, soaked overnight, then boiled in water until soft

1 cup tahini

6 garlic cloves, minced

1 teaspoon cumin

5 tablespoons lemon juice

3 tablespoons olive oil

1 cup water

1. Combine all ingredients in a food processor except water and olive oil.

2. Add the olive oil.

3. Add water little by little until the hummus reaches the desired consistency. You may not use the whole cup.

4. Serve warm or cold.

Lemon Dill Potatoes

This recipe is also good as a variation on typical mashed potato recipes. After boiling the potatoes, mash them. Then add the other ingredients, to taste.

INGREDIENTS | SERVES 4

8 cups potatoes, cubed

Fresh dill, to taste

4 tablespoons freshly squeezed lemon juice

Sea salt, to taste

1. Boil potatoes until soft, approximately 30 minutes.

2. Strain potatoes and place them in a bowl.

3. Gently toss the dill in with the potatoes.

4. Drizzle lemon juice on top, and lightly mix.

5. Add salt, to taste.

How This Supports Your Constitution

White potatoes are not the best choice for vata, though they work for pitta and kapha (if not sweet). The lemon is a nice balance for vata. Even if you serve these potatoes to someone with a vata constitution, you can balance the meal with more supportive foods for vata.

Ginger Lentil Spread

This spread can be eaten in a wrap with added vegetables. It can be spread on pita chips or on vegetables for a satisfying snack.

INGREDIENTS | SERVES 4

½ tablespoon grated ginger

3–5 mushrooms, sliced

2 scallions, sliced

2 tablespoons olive oil

1 tablespoon mustard

2 cups cooked lentils

¼ cup water

Sea salt and pepper, to taste

1. Sauté the ginger, mushrooms, and scallions in olive oil for 5 minutes.

2. Place those ingredients and the remaining ingredients in a food processor.

3. Blend until smooth.

Peanut Sauce

Optional additions to go with this recipe are chili pepper, garlic, or ginger, to taste.

INGREDIENTS | MAKES ABOUT ½ CUP OF SAUCE

¼ cup peanut butter

1 tablespoon tamari

1 tablespoon brown rice vinegar

1 tablespoon maple syrup

¼ cup water

1. With a spoon mix all ingredients in a small pot.

2. Warm the mixture and serve or leave it in the refrigerator overnight to thicken.

CHAPTER 20

Snacks and Desserts

Fun Dessert Crispies

When melting the chocolate, if you melt it in a pot, stir the entire time to prevent it from sticking and burning. Otherwise, use a double boiler.

INGREDIENTS | SERVES 12

4 cups organic puffed rice

1 cup shredded unsweetened coconut

¾ cup melted organic unsweetened chocolate

4 tablespoons almond butter

Maple syrup, to sweeten

1. Mix puffed rice and coconut in a large bowl.

2. Add melted chocolate, almond butter, and maple syrup to the puffed rice mix, and combine.

3. If consistency is too dry, add a few drops of water or unsweetened almond milk.

4. Adjust maple syrup to taste.

5. Spoon mixture into glass baking dish.

6. Refrigerate for 2–4 hours.

Oatmeal Chocolate Cookies

For this tasty recipe, if you cannot find grain-sweetened chocolate chips, you can substitute whatever kind of chocolate chip you'd like. Semisweet is what's typically used for chocolate chip cookies.

INGREDIENTS | MAKES 1 DOZEN COOKIES

1½ cups rolled oats

1 cup whole wheat pastry flour

¼ teaspoon sea salt

½ cup maple syrup

⅓ cup cold-pressed organic sunflower oil or melted, unsalted organic butter, or ghee

1 teaspoon vanilla extract

⅓ cup chopped walnuts or pecans

⅓ cup grain-sweetened chocolate chips

Pouring Love Into Food

Sometimes baking cookies is one of the easiest ways to infuse food with love. Usually you're baking cookies for someone else or for a special occasion, and the love easily flows. Remember that putting that kind of energy into the food you cook is always beneficial whether it's cookies or kale.

1. Preheat oven to 350°F.

2. Combine oats, flour, and salt in a bowl; set aside.

3. In a separate bowl, mix maple syrup, oil (or butter or ghee), and vanilla.

4. Add wet ingredients to dry, and mix well.

5. Stir in nuts and chocolate chips.

6. With moist hands, form dough into balls and flatten slightly.

7. Place on a lightly oiled or lined cookie sheet.

8. Bake on the middle rack for 15–20 minutes until golden on the edges. Keep an eye on the baking time so the chips don't burn.

The Perfect Pecans

This pecan recipe makes pecans so delicious that you can take them as a gift when you go to a friend's house for dinner. They taste perfect on their own, and they are great on salads as a special crunchy treat.

INGREDIENTS | SERVES 6–8

1 egg white
1 teaspoon water
5 cups of whole pecans
½ cup sugar
1 teaspoon cinnamon
¼ teaspoon salt

1. Preheat oven to 225°F.

2. In a large bowl, beat the egg white and water until foamy.

3. Add the pecans to the egg white, and mix until the pecans are coated.

4. In a separate bowl, mix sugar, cinnamon, and salt.

5. Coat the pecans with the dry mixture.

6. Spread the coated pecans on lightly greased cookie sheets.

7. Bake for 1 hour, stirring occasionally; be sure not to burn the pecans.

8. After baking, allow the pecans to cool to room temperature.

Sudha's Heavenly Halva Treats

This one is sure to become a family favorite. It's so quick and simple to make, the kids will be eager to help. This recipe decreases vata and increases pitta and kapha.

INGREDIENTS | SERVES 8

¾ cup tablespoons whole, raw sesame seeds
½ cup sesame tahini
¼ cup honey
½ teaspoon cinnamon
¼ teaspoon salt

1. Dry-roast sesame seeds over low heat until lightly browned. Then let them cool.

2. Grind 8 tablespoons of the seeds with a surabachi mortar and pestle or in a blender.

3. In a medium bowl, combine the tahini, honey, and cinnamon.

4. Add the ground seeds to the tahini mixture and stir until the mix gets very thick; add more crushed seeds if you want a thicker consistency.

5. Form the mixture into small balls about 1 inch in diameter.

6. Combine the salt and remaining 2 tablespoons of whole sesame seeds in a shallow dish.

7. Roll the balls in the sesame seed mix until covered.

8. Let sit a few minutes, then serve. These halva balls can also be made ahead of time and kept in the refrigerator for a cooler snack.

Tofu Cheesecake

Add your favorite seasonal fruits or berries to this recipe for more nutritional value, color, texture, and prana.

INGREDIENTS | MAKES 1 (9-INCH) CHEESECAKE

2 (12-ounce) packages extra firm tofu, drained and cubed

1 cup white sugar

1 teaspoon vanilla extract

¼ teaspoon salt

¼ cup vegetable oil

2 tablespoons lemon juice

1 (9-inch) prepared graham cracker crust

1. In a blender or food processor, combine tofu, sugar, vanilla, salt, vegetable oil, and lemon juice.

2. Blend ingredients until smooth, then pour into piecrust.

3. Bake at 350°F until center is slightly brown, about 20 minutes.

4. Remove from oven to cool.

5. Place in refrigerator until chilled.

Choose Fresh Berries

Get fresh foods every time you can. Fresh, whole foods have *chetana*, which is Sanskrit for "nature's intelligence." Foods that are ripe with nature's intelligence are easier to digest and have more to offer the body and mind than food that has been frozen, processed, or chemically enhanced. Fresh foods are alive with chetana and prana, which your body needs to thrive.

Digestive Chew

Carry this around in your bag or purse, and chew it after meals to help with digestion. It's especially helpful after heavy meals.

INGREDIENTS | **MAKES ENOUGH TO LAST ABOUT 1 MONTH**

⅛ cup cumin seeds

¼ cup fennel seeds

2 teaspoons dill seed (optional)

¼ cup sesame seeds

1. Dry roast the seeds individually in a skillet. Stir them as you roast them for 1–3 minutes, releasing their aromas.

2. Mix them together after they've been dry roasted.

3. Chew about ½ tablespoon after your main meal.

Support Digestion

Insufficient agni (digestive fire) can show up as gas, burping, difficulty waking in the morning, constipation, and body odor. Common ways you may inhibit fire are overeating, grazing, and drinking too much water at meals. To foster good digestion, eat smaller, simpler meals. Sip warm water throughout the day with lemon or lime. Also, try a digestive chew after your meals.

APPENDIX A

Glossary

Abhyanga: herbalized-oil massage

Ahimsa: nonviolence

Allopathic medicine: traditional Western medicine

Ama: undigested substances

Anamaya kosha: food sheath; the densest of five sheaths of the body

Anandamaya kosha: bliss sheath; the subtlest of the five sheaths of the body

Asana: physical posture in hatha yoga practice

Ayurveda: Sanskrit for the science of life, or the science of living. *Ayuh* means "life," and *veda* means "to know," or "knowledge."

Ayurvidya: the living wisdom of Ayurveda. *Ayuh* means "life," and *vidya* means "living wisdom." Ayurvidya is personified as a goddess embodying and transmitting Ayurvedic wisdom.

Chakra: literally means "wheel" or "disc." There are seven major chakras in the body. They are like conductors of energy, and their balance or imbalance affects your overall health.

Chi: the word for life-force energy in Chinese medicine

Constitution: your personal type: how the doshas were set in you when you were conceived

Dhatus: a way of categorizing the tissues and components of the body. There are seven dhatus according to Ayurveda.

Dirgha breath: three-part, or yogic breath

Doshas: literally means "fault" and is used to describe the way that the natural elements are at play in the body and mind. Vata, pitta, and kapha are the three doshas.

Elements: natural energetic forces that support life in nature: ether, air, fire, water, and earth

Gunas: the attributes that apply to everything in the universe, from foods to your mental temperament. *See sattva, tamas, and rajas.*

Hatha yoga: the physical practice of yoga postures

Integrative medicine: draws on complementary systems of health when treating imbalance or disease

Jyotish: Vedic astrology

Kosha: any one of the five sheaths that refer to your physical and energetic bodies

Manomaya Kosha: mental body; one of the five bodies or sheaths

Marma: literally means "vulnerable" or "sensitive." Refers to a place on the body that can be used for healing therapies.

Meditation: the practice of detaching from ongoing trains of thought, or the practice of focusing on a specific object, such as a mantra, image, or candle flame

Mudra: a posture for the hands designed to help direct life-force energy

Nadi: channel in the body that carries energy

Nadi shodhana: an alternate-nostril, channel-purifying, and balancing breath

Panchakarma: literally means "five actions." A practice for purifying the body, helping it release deeply held toxins.

Prakruti: according to Samkya philosophy, the female energy of the universe, creativity/action; your original constitution, how the doshas were arranged in you at conception

Pranamaya kosha: the breath sheath; one of the five bodily sheaths

Pranayama: literally means to control the breath. Breathwork often done as part of a yoga practice.

Purusha: according to Samkya philosophy, pure awareness, the male energy of the universe

Rajas: one of the three gunas. Rajas is associated with movement and passion.

Rasa: the taste of food

Rishi: seer of truth

Samadhi: bliss

Samkya: the philosophy of creation and truth that is the foundation of Ayurveda. The word comes from *sat*, meaning "truth," and *kyah*, meaning "to know."

Sattva: one of the three gunas. It's associated with light, purity, creative potential, and faith.

Savasana: Corpse Pose, relaxation pose

Sushumna: the energy channel that runs up and down the center of the spinal column

Sutra: thread of wisdom, as laid out in the ancient text *Yoga Sutras* by Patanjali

Tamas: one of the three gunas. Characterized by inertia and destructive potential.

Tantu: one of the words that means "pulse"

Tridoshic: the constitution type that is vata-pitta-kapha

Vaidya: Ayurvedic doctor

Vijnanamaya kosha: the wisdom sheath; one of the five sheaths of the body

Vikruti: how the elements are showing up in you now

Vipaka: the postdigestive effect of foods

Virya: the effect a taste has that is warming or cooling to the system

Vishnu mudra: the hand position where the thumb, ring finger, and pinky are extended and the other fingers are bent

Yoga: the union of body, mind, and pure consciousness

Yoga nidra: a practice that invites your awareness through the koshas to the most subtle kosha, where deep relaxation occurs

Whole medical system: a nonspecializing system of health

APPENDIX B

Additional Resources

Books, CDs, DVDs

Arguetty, Danny. *Nourishing the Teacher: Inquiries, Contemplations, & Insights on the Path of Yoga.* (Canada: Danny Arguetty, 2009).

Carlson, Larissa Hall. *Ayurvedic Pranayama and Meditation for the Doshas* [CD]. (Stockbridge, MA: Kripalu Yoga Teachers Association, 2010).

Chödrön, Pema. *Comfortable with Uncertainty.* (Boston, MA: Shambhala, 2002).

Chödrön, Pema. *Taking the Leap.* (Boston, MA: Shambhala, 2009).

Chopra, Deepak. *Journey Into Healing: Awakening the Wisdom Within You.* (New York, NY: Three Rivers Press, 1995).

Chopra, Deepak. *Perfect Health: The Complete Mind Body Guide.* (New York, NY: Harmony, 2001).

Douillard, John. *Perfect Health for Kids: Ten Ayurvedic Health Secrets Every Parent Must Know.* (Berkeley, CA: North Atlantic Books, 2008).

Frawley, David. *Ayurveda and the Mind: The Healing of Consciousness.* (Twin Lakes, WI: Lotus Press, 1996).

Frawley, David. *Yoga and Ayurveda: Self-Healing and Self-Realization.* (Twin Lakes, WI: Lotus Press, 1999).

Frawley, David, Subhash Ranade, and Avinash Lele. *Ayurveda and Marma Therapy: Energy Points in Yogic Healing.* (Twin Lakes, WI: Lotus Press, 2003).

Grilley, Paul. *Chakra Theory and Meditation* [DVD], 2007.

Hirschi, Gertrud. *Mudras: Yoga in Your Hands.* (Newburyport, ME: Weiser Books, 2000).

Judith, Anodea. *Eastern Body Western Mind: Psychology and the Chakra System as a Path to the Self.* (Berkeley, CA: Celestial Arts, 2004).

Judith, Anodea. *The Illuminated Chakras: A Visionary Voyage into Your Inner World* [DVD]. (Llewellyn, 2010).

Lad, Vasant. *Ayurveda: The Science of Self-Healing: A Practical Guide.* (Twin Lakes, WI: Lotus Press, 2009).

Lad, Vasant. *The Complete Book of Ayurvedic Home Remedies.* (New York, NY: Three Rivers Press, 1998).

Lundeen, Sudha Carolyn. *Kripalu Gentle Yoga* [DVD]. (Lenox, MA: Kripalu Center, 2005).

Lundeen, Sudha Carolyn. *Taming the Winds of Vata* [CD]. (Lenox, MA: Kripalu Center, 2011).

Morningstar, Amadea, and Urmila Desai. *The Ayurvedic Cookbook: A Personalized Guide to Good Nutrition and Health.* (Twin Lakes, WI: Lotus Press, 1990).

Pollan, Michael. *In Defense of Food.* (New York, NY: Penguin Press, 2008).

Saraswati, Swami Satyananda. *Yoga Nidra.* (Bihar, India: Yoga Publications Trust, 1998).

Spear, Heidi E. *The Everything® Guide to Chakra Healing: Use Your Body's Subtle Energies to Promote Health, Healing, and Happiness.* (Avon, MA: Adams, 2011).

Svoboda, Robert E. *The Hidden Secret of Ayurveda.* (Albuquerque, NM: The Ayurvedic Press, 2002).

Tiwari, Maya. *A Life of Balance: The Complete Guide to Ayurvedic Nutrition & Body Types, with recipes.* (Rochester, VT: Healing Arts Press, 1995).

Tiwari, Maya. *Living Ahimsa Diet: Nourishing Love & Life.* (Sinking Spring, PA: Mother Om Media, 2011).

Wolfe, David, and Shazzie. *Naked Chocolate.* (San Diego, CA: Maul Brothers, 2005).

Yarema, Thomas, Daniel Rhoda, Johnny Brannigan. *Eat, Taste, Heal: An Ayurvedic Guidebook and Cookbook for Modern Living.* (Kapaa, Hawaii: Five Elements Press, 2006).

Websites

Ayurvedic Institute

The Ayurvedic Institute, recognized as a leading Ayurvedic school and Ayurveda health spa outside of India, was established in 1984 to teach the traditional Ayurvedic medicine of India and to provide these ancient therapies. Ayurvedic healing includes herbs, nutrition, panchakarma cleansing, acupressure massage, yoga, Sanskrit, and Jyotish (Vedic astrology).
www.ayurveda.com

Banyan Botanicals

Banyan Botanicals was founded in 1996, based on the dream of creating a company that would provide the best in Ayurvedic herbs and products, excellent service and guaranteed satisfaction, education, inspiration, and motivation to those seeking greater health and well-being.
www.banyanbotanicals.com

The Boulders Spa

Offers Ayurvedic bodywork, yoga classes, use of an outdoor labyrinth, and more to help you restore balance and well-being.
www.theboulders.com/golden_door_spa/

Chocolate Springs

Specializing in handcrafted European-style gourmet chocolates, as well as homemade ice creams and sorbets.
www.chocolatesprings.com

Chopra Center

Provides daily inspiration, workshops, and resources for healthy living and emotional healing. Online, you'll find a dosha quiz, opportunities for training, and much more.
www.chopra.com

Developmental Delay Resources

The one resource network integrating conventional and holistic approaches for parents and professionals who support children with special needs.
www.devdelay.org

Goldthread Apothecary

An herbal dispensary, farm, and store that sells various products including beautifully combined medicinal loose teas and other natural remedies.
www.goldthreadapothecary.com

Janna Delgado, Ayurvedic Lifestyle Consultant

Offering consultations, programs, and retreats to support and guide you toward health and overall well-being
www.JannaDelgado.com

Kripalu Center for Yoga & Health

Kripalu Center for Yoga & Health is an invaluable resource for books, DVDs, CDs, gemstones, Ayurvedic products, and more. As the nation's largest retreat center for yoga and health, you will find daily classes and workshops, as well as weekend and weeklong programs with internationally known presenters and teachers. Visit the website for information on Kripalu's workshops, School of Ayurveda, bodywork offerings, and products.
www.kripalu.org

Kripalu Professional Associations

Find a trained Ayurvedic or yoga teacher near you. If you are a yoga teacher, join the Kripalu Yoga Teacher's Association for newsletters and a supportive community of other like-minded individuals.
www.kripalu.org/be_a_part_of_kpa/1178

Larissa Carlson

Larissa offers inspirational quotes, workshops, classes, and CDs to support your yoga and Ayurveda journey.
www.larissacarlson.com

NAMA—National Ayurvedic Medical Association

NAMA is the voice of the Ayurvedic community that empowers individuals, communities, and humanity to achieve health and well-being through Ayurveda.
www.ayurvedanama.org

Nourish Your Light

Nourish Your Light strives to offer resources and services that facilitate self-discovery, unearth inner wisdom, and awaken the art of living yoga.
www.nourishyourlight.com

Organic India

Organic India means absolute commitment to quality. All their products are 100 percent organic, pure, and natural because you want the best for your family and so do they. The guiding principles of this company are health and happiness for all beings and great respect for the Divine Mystery of Mother Nature, who selflessly sustains humanity and naturally provides us all with a bounty of nourishing foods and healing herbs.
www.OrganicIndia.com

Planet Sark

A resource for inspiration, supporting your creative dreams.
www.planetsark.com

Practice Your Joy

Learn ways to use yoga, Ayurvedic principles, Shakespeare, chocolate, and more to live more often in your blissful center. Enjoy your practice, practice your joy.
www.PracticeYourJoy.com

Sarada Ayurvedic Remedies

Centuries-old Ayurvedic formulas with the finest herbs, minerally rich purified clays, and naturally processed oils that gently cleanse and nourish all types.
www.saradausa.com

Sudha Carolyn Lundeen, RN, RYT-500

A certified holistic-health nurse, Ayurvedic health and lifestyle coach, workshop leader, yoga instructor/therapist, and senior Kripalu teacher, Sudha leads 200- and 500-hour Kripalu yoga teacher trainings and is on the faculty of the Kripalu School of Ayurveda. She leads workshops internationally and is the creator of the newly released CD *Taming the Winds of Vata* and the award-winning DVD *Kripalu Gentle Yoga*.
www.sudhalundeen.com

Index

W

Y

We Have
EVERYTHING®
on Anything!

With more than 19 million copies sold, **the Everything® series** has become one of America's favorite resources for solving problems, learning new skills, and organizing lives. Our brand is not only recognizable—it's also welcomed.

The series is a hand-in-hand partner for people who are ready to tackle new subjects—like you!

For more information on the Everything® series, please visit *www.adamsmedia.com*

The Everything® list spans a wide range of subjects, with more than 500 titles covering 25 different categories:

Business	History	Reference
Careers	Home Improvement	Religion
Children's Storybooks	Everything Kids	Self-Help
Computers	Languages	Sports & Fitness
Cooking	Music	Travel
Crafts and Hobbies	New Age	Wedding
Education/Schools	Parenting	Writing
Games and Puzzles	Personal Finance	
Health	Pets	